An A-Z Woman's Guide to Vibrant Health

Prevent and Treat the Top 25 Female Health Conditions

D0968076

An A-Z Woman's Guide to Vibrant Health

Prevent and Treat the Top 25 Female Health Conditions

Lorna R. Vanderhaeghe

Health Venture Publications

First published in Canada in 2004 by Health Venture Publications

1 2 3 4 5 QCE 08 07 06 05 04

ISBN: 0-9734297-2-0

Cover photograph by Donna Newman
Lorna Vanderhaeghe with daughters Caitlyn and Crystal
Cover and book design by Sam Truax and BbM Graphics
Edited by Susan Girvan

DISCLAIMER: While all care is taken with the accuracy of the facts and procedures in this book, the author accepts neither liability nor responsibility to any person with respect to loss, injury or damage caused, or alleged to be caused directly or indirectly, by the information contained in this book. The purpose of this book is to educate and inform. For medical advice you should seek the individual, personal advice and services of a health care professional.

Those wishing to obtain additional copies of this book or requesting permission to reproduce material from it may contact:

Health Venture Publications
5948 3rd Line R.R. #1
Hillsburgh, ON   N0B 1Z0

Printed and bound in Canada

I dedicate this book to women of all ages.

Women constitute 53% of the earth's population. They perform two-thirds of the world's work for which they earn 10% of the income. They own 1% of the property and they have 100% of the children. Given these statistics, women should hold the majority of the political power in the world.

– *Helen Caldicott, M.D., pediatrician, anti-nuclear activist, author of* If You Love This Planet

We don't because we are too tired from
looking after our families, jobs and homes.

CONTENTS

INTRODUCTION

How would you describe the state of your health? Do you wish you could say it was "vibrant"?

During my years of research into alternative medicine to help my friends and family with their health—now more than twenty—and after talking to thousands of women, I know that many women do not feel well, let alone "vibrant." In fact, given the information that's surfacing in the media, I would say that women's health is under siege. Statistics in both Canada and the U.S. tell the same story.

- **Heart Disease:** Women's rates of heart disease are now equal to men's, but more women die of heart attacks. This is the number one cause of death of women of all ages.

- **Breast Cancer:** In 1960, one in 20 women developed breast cancer; today that figure is one in eight. In fact, breast cancer is the leading cause of death in women between the ages of 35 and 54.

- **Obesity:** Over 50 percent of women are overweight, and of these, 30 percent are dangerously obese. While obesity is rarely listed on death certificates, this "un-indicted" killer leads to countless health problems: Type 2 diabetes, greater risk for breast cancer, heart disease and stroke, as well as arthritis, asthma, depression and sleep apnea.

- **Osteoporosis:** One in four women have osteoporosis. Of those with an osteoporosis-related hip fracture, 20 percent will die; another 20 percent will never get out of long-term care facilities.

- **Cervical Cancer:** Death rates from cervical cancer are highest in women over the age of 50 because these women often fail to have annual PAP tests once they are post-menopausal. The number of women with Human Papilloma Virus induced abnormal cervical cells (a risk factor for cervical cancer) is skyrocketing, yet fifteen percent of North American women have never had a PAP test. And over 30 percent of women have not had a PAP test in the last three years.

■ **Stress:** Stress and its negative effects on the body have surpassed the common cold as the most prevalent health problem in North America. If you are one of those women who is doing laundry at midnight and then up at 6 a.m. to start another non-stop day, be aware that at some point, if the pace of your life—and the stress that accompanies it—is not reduced, your body will say "no more." It will do this by being physically overwhelmed by all the abuse it's taking, and letting disease take hold.

In the midst of taking care of your family, your company and perhaps the rest of the world, ask yourself, "Who is taking care of me?" You may need to re-evaluate what needs to be done (and who else could do it), learn to control the emotions that put you into a negative spiral and blind you to all the positive things in your life or simply say, "No, I can't take that on."

Aside from the conditions mentioned above, modern women are plagued with hormonal problems, including severe menstrual cramps, PMS, endometriosis, uterine fibroids, ovarian cysts, infertility, heavy periods and urinary tract infections to name a few. I deal with these health conditions and more in the core of this book. Each condition is defined and probable causes and common symptoms are given. My goal is to present you with alternatives to synthetic hormones and other drug treatments. I provide the alternatives, along with the food supplement suggestions in the form of a "Prescription for Health," followed by "Health Tips to Enhance Healing," to give you everything you need to know to obtain vibrant health.

The "Prescription for Health" recommends only researched supplements. Most of these supplements have either double-blind, placebo-controlled, clinical studies or decades of use to back up their reputations. It is important that you use nutrients that have been scientifically validated. The effects of many prescription drugs have never been researched by testing on women; I tried to find nutritional supplements that have had their efficacy proven in females.

When following the supplement recommendations in one of my prescriptions, start with those at the top of the list. You will notice that every condition requires a multivitamin with minerals and essential fatty acids. You will also note that some conditions need several supplements. Most of those are sold in multi-ingredient formulas so, although it may look daunting to take six nutrients, you will actually only be taking only one formula along with your multivitamin with minerals.

Something else I've learned after two decades of writing and lecturing: many of the nutrients I wanted to recommend were not readily available. After thousands of letters and requests from people, I decided to formulate a line of nutritional supplements that were high quality, free of allergens and included clinically proven ingredients. Furthermore, it was important to me to provide third-party verification of the ingredients so that people would be guaranteed that what they were buying was actually in the supplement. Some of the supplements recommended here will be from my own line, while others are from companies that I feel have top-quality formulators who use science as the foundation for their excellent nutrients.

Contrary to what some nutritionists and medical doctors insist, you cannot get all of your nutrients from the food you eat. While a healthy diet and regular exercise are essential to good health, few of us manage to achieve even those basics. And even if you do eat a varied diet of organic fruits and vegetables (seven to ten half-cup servings), wild fish, organic meats and poultry, whole grains and healthy fats *and* you drink plenty of clean water every day, there will be nutrient deficiencies in your diet. Our environment is polluted, and many of the foods we eat have been harvested before they are ripe, grown in soils that are exhausted of essential elements, and stripped of their nutrients during processing.

If you consume the standard North American diet (no breakfast, convenience foods, snacks filled with fake sugars and trans-fatty acids, few vegetables or fruits, meats and dairy products loaded with hormones and lots of coffee or sodas), you must take a good foundation supplement of multivitamins with minerals.

I have seen the healing benefits of a complete multi-nutrient program in the health of my friends, family and readers. Fuel your body with the right nutrients, and you will be helping your body fend off disease and protect itself from the effects of stress, and supporting its efforts to rid itself of the chemicals we are exposed to daily.

I have tried to simplify the mass of information and suggestions for vibrant health and make them easy to adopt. The final step is up to you—too many women intend to take their supplements every day, but forget. Put the bottle on the kitchen table so you remember to take them with your food every day. Better yet—dish them out when you feed the entire family.

As a woman over forty with two daughters (my oldest is mother of three children), I know how important multi-nutrients are to our health. Nutrients aren't optional—they are essential. They ensure that our hearts stay strong well into our nineties, that our breasts are protected from disease, that our thyroids function properly and that our bones don't crumble. I've created this book to educate and empower you so that you will no longer suffer from many of the common health conditions (or the treatments that often go with them). As women become more educated, I trust we will demand better diagnostic procedures and treatments that "first do no harm" as they ease the suffering. The first step is for you to become an active participant in maintaining your health.

—*Lorna Vanderhaeghe*

PS: I have included some Self-Assessment Questionnaires and information about standard diagnostic tests and treatments in the appendices of this book. The more knowledge you have when you enter your physician's office, the better your treatment outcome will be.

References for the information in this book will be posted on my web site at www.hormonehelp.com, along with detailed information on each nutritional formula recommended in the book.

Health Conditions

ACNE (hormonal)

During puberty, peri-menopause and menopause sebaceous (oil) glands become more active. Pores can become clogged with sebum, dried skin and bacteria, causing skin to erupt into pimples, red blotches and sometimes inflamed and infected abscesses. Acne normally appears on the face, shoulders, scalp, upper arms and legs, upper chest and back. More than 40 percent of teens seek treatment from a specialist for their acne condition.

Hormonal acne break-outs tend to occur during ovulation or the week before menstruation. In those women with hormonally induced acne, when the ovary releases the egg, it often is not able to completely release it. When this occurs, androgens (male hormones) are secreted in excess and women develop acne around the hair line, chin and chest and back. To correct hormonal acne many doctors prescribe birth control pills to stop ovulation. (Today we have 12-year- olds on birth control pills to control acne.) Nutritional supplements can normalize ovulation and eliminate the problem at the source. Even mild episodes of acne can lead to scarring, and scars can be both physical and psychological.

Symptoms

There are various types of skin lesions: a *papule* is a round bump that may be invisible but makes the skin feel rough like sandpaper. A *comedo* occurs when an oil follicle becomes plugged with oil, dead skin, tiny hairs or bacteria. An *open comedo* is known as a blackhead, and a *closed comedo* is commonly referred to as a whitehead. The temporary red or pink spot after an acne lesion has healed is referred to as a *macule*, and several together contribute to the appearance of inflammation associated with acne. A *nodule* is another dome-shaped lesion similar to a papule, but it extends deeper into the skin causing the destruction of tissues that leads to scarring. Nodules can be painful, as can cysts which are filled with liquid, can be severely inflamed and also affect deeper skin layers.

Causes

While food choices have been hotly debated as a cause of acne for years, research out of the University of Colorado is confirming that a diet high in refined carbohydrates permanently boosts insulin and thus promotes acne. According to Dr. Loren Cordain, sustained high insulin levels elevate hormone levels, stimulating the production of oil that leads to clogged pores, bacterial growth and acne. High-glycemic foods such as breads, cakes, sugars and soda are major culprits in acne. Although acne is epidemic in our society, it is virtually unknown in New Guinea and the Amazon where diets focus on fruits and vegetables. Those with acne should be conscious of foods that aggravate the condition. Acne is also associated with low stomach acidity, suggesting incomplete food breakdown and imbalances in the digestive tract.

With the shift between male hormones and female hormones during the menstrual cycle, acne lesions change. Synthetic progestins and estrogens used for menopausal symptoms, supplements of DHEA, endometriosis, polycystic ovarian syndrome and estrogen dominance have been linked to acne. Other drugs such as corticosteroids, anabolic steroids, iodides and bromides are also known to cause acne, as are cosmetics that block pores.

PRESCRIPTION FOR HEALTHY SKIN

Nutrients	Dosage	Action
Multivitamins with minerals (FemmEssentials or MultiEssentials) See Appendix A for complete formula recommendations	As directed; should contain the following nutrients: • Vitamin A 5000 IU • Beta carotene 15000 IU • Folic acid 1 mg • P-5-P (vitamin B6) 60 mg • Vitamin B3 30 mg, along with other B vitamins • Vitamin D 400 IU Promotes healing of skin • Vitamin E 200 IU • Zinc 15 mg per day. In one study 135 mg of zinc daily was as effective as 750 mg daily tetracycline without side effects. • Chromium picolinate 200 mg per day • Selenium 100 mcg	Reduces sebum production, promotes smooth, clear skin Facilitates breaking down of excess hormones Acts as an antioxidant and encourages tissue repair Essential for healthy immune function Improves glucose tolerance and essential fatty acid metabolism To enhance glutathione and fight bacteria

Evening Primrose or Borage oil	1000 mg per day	Helps fight acne
Omega-3 Fatty Acids	1000 mg Pharmaceutical grade fish oil	Helps heal skin
EstroSense	2 capsules per day containing: • Indole-3-carbinol 150 mg • Sulforaphane 200 mcg • Calcium D-glucarate 150 mg • Curcumin 50 mg • Milk thistle 50 mg • Rosemary 25 mg • Green tea extract 100 mg • Lycopene 5 mg	Balances hormones supports healthy ovulation. Within two menstrual cycles acne will clear and PMS, period problems will ease.
BB536 Bifidobacterium	2 capsules daily, containing 2.5 billion active cells	Improves intestinal flora (especially important if you have taken antibiotics for condition)
Garlic	eat foods containing garlic	Acts as a natural antibacterial
Artichoke	160-320 mg three times daily with meals, assuming standardized to contain 13-18% caffeolquinic acids calculated as chlorogenic acid	Increases bile formation and flow to digest and absorb fats
Chaste Tree Berry (Vitex)	As directed	Normalizes hormones
Dandelion Root	Dandelion tea as a beverage	Detoxifies the liver
Digestive enzymes (Zymactive)	1 or 2 capsules with meals	Aids digestion

HEALTH TIPS TO ENHANCE HEALING

■ Wash gently with warm water and an irritant-free cleanser. Avoid scrubbing, which can stimulate sebum production. Do not use make-up that will clog pores.

■ Do not pick at acne, as this can lead to infection.

- If you have gas, bloating, indigestion or constipation, you have low stomach acid. Add a supplement with betaine hydrochloride or digestive enzymes to improve digestion.
- Avoid the use of antibiotics which can cause *Candida* yeast overgrowth and vaginal infections which will worsen acne symptoms in the long term and may have little effect on the acne.
- Focus on a diet rich in fruits and vegetables along with 25 g of fiber to help naturally eliminate estrogen. Avoid foods that you know aggravate the condition.
- Treat constipation. Holding days of toxic waste increases the amount of toxins excreted by the skin. *See* Constipation.

Adrenal Exhaustion

The adrenal glands get very little attention in western medicine, yet they have the important job of secreting sex hormones and stress hormones that guide reactions to a stressor throughout the entire body. We have two adrenal glands, which are comprised of two parts: the *medulla* and the *cortex*. The medulla triggers the instinctual "flight or fight" response, including the increase of blood sugar levels, the rate of breathing, cardiac output and blood flow to the brain, lungs and muscles. The cortex produces hormones that are essential in regulating excretory, immune defense, metabolic, mineral balancing and reproductive functions. The cortex also secretes corticosteroids in response to stress, and these hormones help us to cope with long-term stressors by converting protein to energy. This energy remains available long after the "flight or fight" response subsides. Adrenal exhaustion occurs when the glands wear out from the continual production of the stress hormone cortisol, and can lead to Chronic Fatigue Syndrome and eventually Addison's disease. Most importantly adrenal exhaustion promotes hormone imbalance. The adrenal glands and the thyroid are linked. If the adrenals become stressed, the thyroid gland can produce less thyroid hormone and vice versa. Most people today, particularly women, have some degree of compromised adrenal gland function due to stressful lives.

Symptoms
Extreme hot flashes and night sweats, insomnia (you go to bed but three hours later you are wide awake), environmental sensitivities, hypoglycemia, poor

concentration, low energy, dizziness upon rising, irritability, nervousness or anxiety, shortness of breath, knee problems, muscle twitching, heart palpitations, sensitivity to light, digestive problems or cravings for salt, sugar, junk food or coffee.

To test your adrenal gland function, rest for five minutes and then take your blood pressure. Stand up, and immediately take another blood pressure reading. If the reading is lower when you are standing than when you are resting, you can suspect decreased adrenal gland function.

Causes

Sustained periods of high stress lead to chronic elevation of the stress hormone cortisol, which research now links to bone loss, compromised immune function, chronic fatigue, exhaustion, fat accumulation, infertility and memory loss. During menopause, the workload of the adrenals also increases as these glands are a primary source of sex hormones, including estrogen.

For women, particularly those who come home from a full-time job to care for their families, cortisol remains elevated in the evening when it naturally should subside to allow the onset of sleep.

PRESCRIPTION FOR HEALTH

Nutrients	Dosage	Action
Multivitamins with minerals (FemmEssentials or MultiEssentials)	As directed. See Appendix A for the complete listing of recommended nutrients and their actions.	Provides all the nutrients a woman needs every day to support all functions
Rhodiola (Rhodiola rosea)	100 mg one to three times daily	Helps reduce the effects of stress, is anti-aging and regulates the heart by increasing oxygen utilization
Suma (Pfaffia Paniculata)	100 mg one to three times daily	A regenerative tonic used for nervous, reproductive, hormonal and digestive disorders

Ashwagandha (Withana somnifera)	80 mg one to three times daily	Improves energy, supports the immune system, is anti-oxidant, anti-inflammatory, improves sexual performance. It is also used to aid conversion of T4 to T3 thyroid hormone
Siberian Ginseng (Eleutherococcus senticosus)	100 mg one to three times daily (Siberian ginseng is not a true ginseng)	Normalizes reactions to physical and mental stress, enhances energy, protects against environmental pollutants, regulates blood sugar, protects the liver and adrenals
Schizandra berries (Schizandra chinensis)	80 mg one to three times daily	For insomnia, nervousness, supports the liver, improves physical endurance
Evening Primrose or Borage oil	1000 mg per day	Supports nervous system
Omega-3 Fatty Acids	1000 mg pharmaceutical grade fish oil	Helps protect the cardio-vascular and nervous system

HEALTH TIPS TO FIGHT STRESS

- Breathing is a powerful de-stressing tool. Several times per day, breathe in through your nose and fill your lungs with air until your abdomen rises. Then slowly exhale from your mouth until your lungs are empty. Repeat this five times.
- Get eight hours of sleep every night and try to sleep until 7:30 in the morning.
- Just say "no" when you have too much to accomplish in one day.
- Share the household workload with family.
- Eat seven to 10 half-cup servings of fruits and vegetables every day.
- Smile. Purge negative emotions such as anger and hatred.
- Get help in dealing with grief. The loss of a loved one, a divorce, or the loss of a job all produce grief. Immune suppression is the result when grief is not dealt with.
- *Carpe diem*–seize the day–and live it to the fullest. Don't worry so much about tomorrow.

- Believe in yourself. Negative self-talk and continually doubting your abilities hamper your body's ability to heal.
- See the beauty around you. Smell the flowers, watch the sunset and listen to the wind.
- Love your family and friends, and be forgiving.
- Be good to yourself. Most of us are our own worst enemies. We focus on our weaknesses and minimize our strengths. Wake up each day and tell yourself you are a good and useful person.
- Do the things you have always wanted to do. Learn to water ski, sing in a choir, write a book, tell stories to your grandchildren, walk, garden–whatever makes you happy.
- Seek your spiritual side. This does not have to be religious, although those with strong religious beliefs generally live at peace and feel protected. Most of us believe in something greater than ourselves, a spiritual power that offers solace and helps us find the quiet place within.
- Take AdrenaSense containing rhodiola, suma, ashwagandha, ginseng and schizandra.

Anemia

There are several types of anemia whereby the number of red blood cells, or the amount of hemoglobin they carry, is low. A reduction of either limits the amount of oxygen available to the lungs and other areas of the body. A simple blood test can determine anemia.

Iron-deficiency anemia is the most common type. When red blood cells are lost due to excessive bleeding, a deficiency of iron occurs. Normally iron is recycled to make new red blood cells, but when excess bleeding has occurred (often due to uterine fibroids in women) there is not enough iron to rebuild red blood cells in the bone marrow. Iron supplements are used with success to correct iron-deficiency anemia.

Vitamin B12 and folic acid are also used by the bone marrow to make red blood cells. A deficiency of one or both causes *pernicious anemia*. Vegetarians, and those with malabsorption syndromes caused by gut problems or autoimmune disease such as Crohn's or autoimmune gastritis, must use Vitamin B12 and folic acid injections to correct this anemia.

Vitamin C deficiency causes small red blood cells; this condition also promotes anemia.

Pernicious anemia is associated with autoimmune disease. It develops at the last stage of autoimmune gastritis because the immune system has destroyed the gastric mucosa (gut lining). Autoimmune hemolytic anemia results when red blood cells are attacked and destroyed. The body is unable to use Vitamin B12 and as a result, digestion is compromised, as is the body's ability to produce red blood cells. Ten to 15 percent of those with autoimmune gastritis have pernicious anemia.

Two percent of the Western population over 60 years of age is deficient in vitamin B12 and has pernicious anemia. Pernicious anemia can easily be treated with vitamin B12.

Symptoms
Signs of anemia are fatigue, shortness of breath, depression, diarrhea, paleness, rapid heartbeat, chest pains, inability to exercise even moderately and abdominal discomfort. Stomach acid is extremely low, making digestion difficult or impossible. Iron deficiency can cause craving for dirt and ice. Cracks at the sides of the mouth and spoonlike fingernails are also signs of anemia. If vitamin B12 deficiency is left unaddressed, neurological problems can arise. Many elderly people have undiagnosed B12 and folic acid deficiencies, leading to anemia.

Causes
The cause of pernicious anemia is still unknown, but two factors are acknowledged. First, there is a genetic inheritance leaning towards northern Europeans and those with genetic markers for fair skin, blue eyes and blood group A. It is very rare in southern Europeans and "almost nonexistent" in Asians and Africans. Second, it coexists with other autoimmune disorders such as Hashimoto's thyroiditis, primary Addison's disease, Type 1 diabetes, vitiligo, myasthenia gravis, premature graying and primary ovarian failure. A lack of intrinsic factor needed to absorb B12 is often the cause of pernicious anemia. (Intrinsic factor is secreted

by the cells of the stomach; these cells are often damaged due to disease. Or intrinsic factor may not be released due to low levels of stomach acid and the pancreatic enzyme trypsin.)

Vitamin B12 deficiency can be caused by poor nutrition, a strict vegetarian or vegan diet, or any digestive disorder such as malabsorption syndrome, Crohn's disease, leaky gut or gastric surgery.

PRESCRIPTION FOR HEALTH

Nutrient	Dosage	Action
Multivitamins with minerals (FemmEssentials or MultiEssentials)	As directed. For complete formula recommendations see Appendix A	For optimal nutrient status
Vitamin B12	Injection 1 mg weekly for 6 weeks or until anemia is reversed, then once monthly. Those with pernicious anemia need B12 for life. Oral methylcobalamin, the active form of B12 in sublingual tablets 2000 mcg per day for one month or until anemia is reversed and 1000 mcg thereafter.	Essential for blood cell formation
Folic Acid	1000 mcg daily	Required for blood cell formation
Lipotropic factors Choline and inositol	100 mg Choline daily 100 mg inositol daily	Maximizes assimilation of B12
Vitamin B6 from Pyridoxal-5-phosphate	50 mg per day	Elevates hemoglobin

Vitamin C	1000 mg three times daily	Maximizes assimilation of B12 and eliminates iron-deficiency anemia
Floradix Iron Tonic	1-4 capfuls daily	Does not constipate, enhances iron
Lactobacillus Acidophilus	1 teaspoon, 1-2 billion active organisms daily	Improves intestinal flora required to manufacture nutrients
Digestive enzymes (Zymactive)	1-2 capsules with meals	Maximizes digestion

HEALTH TIPS TO ENHANCE HEALING

- Uterine fibroids are a common cause of abnormal menstrual bleeding in women. *See* Uterine Fibroids for treatment information.
- Avoid alcohol, coffee, tobacco, birth control pills and topical steroids—they inhibit vitamin B12 absorption.
- Take digestive enzymes before a meal, but do not drink fluids while eating—that will dilute digestive enzymes.
- Eat calf liver.
- Eat plenty of dark green leafy vegetables.
- Lack of iron inhibits thyroid hormone. Have your thyroid checked.

Arthritis

Millions of people suffer from one form of arthritis or another and, contrary to popular belief, it is not a disease affecting only the elderly. Some forms of arthritis strike toddlers, while thousands are stricken in the prime of their lives. Arthritis is the most prevalent chronic condition affecting women, particularly between the ages of 20 and 40. The National Institute of Arthritis and Musculoskeletal and Skin Diseases reports that one in seven persons have some form of arthritis.

Arthritis ("arth" meaning joint, "itis" meaning inflammation) consists of over 100 different conditions from gout to rheumatoid arthritis (see box for a partial list). Although most of these disorders occur with joint or muscle inflammation, many, like lupus, involve the skin, lungs and kidney. Inflammation, swelling and, most importantly, pain, are hallmarks of arthritis.

Osteoarthritis, the most common form of arthritis, is a gradual wearing away of the cartilage that cushions the joints and prevents the bones from scraping against each other. New research is also finding that osteoarthritis occurs when the ability to regenerate normal cartilage is impaired. Repetitive activities and sports injuries are associated with the development of arthritis.

Rheumatoid arthritis (RA), the second most common form, is an autoimmune disease whereby the immune system produces antibodies that destroy the synovial membranes around the lubricating fluid in the joints. RA may begin in fits and starts, taking months or years to progress, but for about 25 percent of sufferers it begins abruptly and severely. In the case of RA, correcting the immune system abnormality is the focus of treatment.

TYPES OF ARTHRITIS

- Ankylosing Spondylitis
- Gout
- Systemic Lupus Erythematosus
- Osteoarthritis
  (the most common type)
- Polymyalgia Rheumatica
- Pseudo Gout

- Psoriatic Arthritis
- Raynaud's Phenomenon
- Juvenile Chronic Arthritis
- Reiter's Disease
- Rheumatoid Arthritis
- Infective Arthritis
- Sjogren's Syndrome

Symptoms
Osteoarthritis: Usually osteoarthritis appears after the age of forty and is characterized by joint pain and stiffness that increases in severity over a long period of time. The joints become swollen and lose their mobility. After much of the cartilage has been worn away, bone spurs develop in the joint spaces.

Rheumatoid Arthritis: The joint pain and stiffness of RA is more noticeable in the morning and, like osteoarthritis, the joints become swollen. Unlike osteoarthritis, however, RA can strike suddenly in some cases and at any time of life, even in childhood (Juvenile Rheumatoid Arthritis). Other symptoms include fatigue, fever, depression, anemia, weight loss and night sweats. When the joints are inflamed they take on a purplish color and, as the disease progresses, the hands and feet become deformed. RA attacks symmetrically, afflicting both wrists, ankles or both knees.

When diagnosing RA, four out of seven criteria must be met: morning stiffness that lasts more than an hour; the arthritis is symmetrical; three joint areas simultaneously inflamed (not just bony overgrowth); arthritis is present in any of the hand joints; nodules lay under the skin on bony prominences; serum rheumatoid factor levels are abnormal; and erosions or decalcification are detected by X-ray.

Causes
Osteoarthritis: Better known as "wear and tear" arthritis, as the nickname suggests, it can arise from repetitive use or abuse of the joints from heavy labor, sports and injuries. Obesity aggravates arthritis because greater strain is put on the joints. Poor nutrition and dehydration as well as food and environmental allergies can contribute to the condition. Although aging is usually cited as a factor (70 percent of the elderly have it), there is an assumption that it is an inevitable aspect of aging. This is not true. If care is taken to address the other factors, then you may live a long life without osteoarthritis.

Rheumatoid Arthritis: Stress and its ability to affect hormones that promote inflammation, allergies, heredity, obesity, nutritional deficiencies, vaccines, a hyperactive immune system and even viral or bacterial infections are just a few of the potential causes of RA. Ten years ago rheumatologists would have disagreed that these factors play a role in promoting arthritis, but new research has shown otherwise.

PRESCRIPTION FOR HEALTH
There are many nutrients clinically researched for the treatment of arthritis. You may want to try Celadrin and ArthriSense first. ArthriSense contains most of the ingredients listed below it.

Nutrient	Dosage	Action
Multivitamin with minerals (FemmEssentials or MultiEssentials)	As directed. See Appendix A for complete list of nutrients suggested	Supports all body systems including cardiovascular, nervous, hormonal, and endocrine systems, bones and more
Celadrin, both oral and topical	1500 mg per day Topical apply twice per day	Anti-inflammatory, reduces pain and swelling of joints
ArthriSense both oral and topical Containing bosweilla, white willow bark, yucca root, Devil's claw, sarsaparilla, feverfew and bromelain	2 capsules 2 times daily Topical apply twice per day	Reduces joint pain and swelling, speeds repair of cartilage. Is anti-inflammatory
Omega-3 essential fatty acids	Fish oil pharmaceutical grade 3000 mg per day	Is a potent anti-inflammtory and improves mobility
Glucosamine Sulfate	Take 500 mg three times daily	For cartilage repair
Green-lipped muscle (a rich source of glycosaminoglycans)	As directed	Building block of cartilage
MSM	1 to 2 grams daily	Anti-inflammatory
GLA Evening Primrose or borage Oil	1000 to 2000 mg per day	Relieves pain and inflammation
Zymactive	As directed on bottle	*See* Bromelain below
SAM-e S-adenosyl-methionine	200 mg twice daily	Sulfur compound that reduces pain and inflammation; promotes proteoglycan production

DHEA	Have a DHEAS test by your doctor to see if you are deficient. 5-10 mg per day DHEA (In Canada it is available through the drug release program prescribed by your doctor)	Reduces IL-6, normalizes cortisol and stops inflammatory processes
Bromelain	Take 2000 to 6000 mcu (1300 to 4000 gdu) on an empty stomach.	Contains enzymes, anti-inflammatory, improves joint mobility, reduces swelling
Boswellia	Standardized dose of 400 mg, three times per day	Anti-inflammatory as effective as NSAIDS
Devil's Claw	1 to 2 grams of standardized Devil's Claw should be taken daily	Anti-inflammatory
Feverfew	(standardized to .6% parthenolides)	Suppresses prostaglandin production, eases pain and inflammation
Turmeric	Three 400-mg doses per day	Anti-inflammatory
Willow Bark	Standardized willow bark is available; dosages range from 200 mg to 1000 mg	Reduces pain and inflammation

HEALTH TIPS TO ENHANCE HEALING

- Drink 8 to 10 glasses of pure, clean water every day to prevent your joint cushions from becoming dehydrated. For every juice or caffeine beverage that you consume, you must have another glass of water.
- Avoid these substances to prevent flare-ups: citrus fruit, milk, red meat, sugar products, salt, paprika and cayenne pepper, tobacco and any member of the nightshade family (potatoes, eggplant, tomatoes, peppers, etc.).
- Focus your diet on natural, whole foods: fresh fruit, vegetables, legumes, eggs, whole grains, healthy fats and oils, seafood and fresh fish. They are key to halting inflammation at the source. Eat foods with a high sulfur content that

will help remove metals from the body including garlic, onions and asparagus.

- Non-weight bearing exercise like water aerobics, swimming, stationary cycling and yoga should be performed. Be careful not to overburden joints or cause pain and inflammation.
- Lose weight. Even 10 extra pounds can cause an additional 40 pounds of pressure on arthritic knee and ankle joints.

Other Recommendations

- Use hot or cold compresses on the area to alleviate pain and inflammation. Take hot baths or saunas to keep the joints warm.
- Use topical ointments including ArthriSense and Celadrin. Look for products that contain capsaicin, dimethyl sulfoxide (DMSO) or quaternary amines. Look for capsaicin creams containing 0.025 to 0.075 percent capsaicin (avoid contact with eyes)
- Start a diet diary and write down everything you eat to see if there is any correlation to your arthritis symptoms. Ask for a referral to an allergy specialist and get tested for possible triggers. Some allergies may only be detected with the help of an ELISA test. Once you know what you are allergic to, avoid those allergens.
- Beware of taking nonsteroidal anti-inflammatory drugs (NSAIDs), Celebrex and Acetaminophen long term due to gut problems.

Health Fact

If you are taking methotrexate, you must supplement with B vitamins and folic acid as the drug reduces these nutrients, promoting nausea and diarrhea. Pernicious anemia develops if not addressed.

Breast Cancer

Breast cancer is the primary cause of death for women between the ages of 35 and 54. Despite great strides in our medical knowledge, cancer rates have increased dramatically in the last 40 years. In 1960, one in 20 women developed breast cancer. Today, that number is one in eight. Sadly, one quarter of women who develop breast cancer will die from the disease.

Normal healthy cells go through a series of steps to ensure life. They grow, divide, and die in a carefully performed, predetermined symphony. During this highly complex process, the cell's genetic code of DNA is duplicated and transferred to new cells. Normally this process takes place without error, but every once in a while a mistake occurs. Most mistakes are quickly repaired, but on occasion a mistake may not be detected and cells will be allowed to perform differently than usual. Normal cell conduct organizes cells into their correct location, turns growth off and on as required, and ensures that cells do not crowd each other.

Cancer cells do not play by the rules. Cancer begins in normal cells that have become renegades. These abnormal cells, also called *malignant cells*, turn the immune system against itself, multiply unchecked, steal nutrients, re-route blood supplies away from normal body functions and lack preprogrammed cell death (called apoptosis). Because these turncoat cells are similar to other healthy cells, often the immune system fails to detect and kill them. The cancer cells' goal is to survive at all cost, even if they kill their host. The key to stopping breast cancer is to determine what triggers abnormal cell reproduction and put an end to it.

Symptoms

Early detection of breast cancer is crucial. Become familiar with the look and feel of your breasts, and report any changes to your doctor. According to the National Cancer institute, nipple tenderness, discharge or nipples turning in toward the breast should be reported. Any lump or thickness located in or near the breast and under the arm, or a change in the size or shape of the breast is cause for concern. Breasts are lumpy by nature, so do not panic if you locate a lump. Benign lumps tend to be soft, smooth, round and movable, while cancerous lumps are firmly attached within the breast and tend to be hard, with an odd shape. Talk to your doctor if the skin on your areola, nipple or breast is red, scaly, or swollen with ridges or dimpling like an orange peel.

Mammography is a method for finding lumps, but it has its limitations (*see* mammography, MRI and thermography in Appendix C). For women under the age of 40, mammograms are difficult to interpret due to denser breast tissue, benign or fibrocystic breast disease. Mammograms are also unreliable, often giving false positive and false negative readings. Mammography ranges from being uncomfortable to being downright painful for women, and exposure to the radiation with each successive test increases breast cancer risk.

Breast thermography and MRI are safe alternatives to mammography. Any suspicious lumps receive a biopsy, which involves the removal of tissue with a needle. This procedure confirms or rules out the diagnosis of cancer.

Causes

Defects in the genetic code of the cell are not the sole cause of cancer; when these defects are combined with environmental and lifestyle factors including the use of hormones, pesticides, radiation, stress, toxic agents, viruses and nutritional deficiencies, cancer cells get the green light. Since most of these factors are controllable, we need to define the external factors that increase our risk of breast cancer.

According to Dr. Susan Love, author of *Breast Book*, breast cancer may be caused by a combination of genes that are mutated by cancer-causing agents known as carcinogens. Carcinogens cause uncontrolled cell growth that is strictly confined to the ductal or lobular units of the breast, and these growths are known as *precancerous lesions*. With additional mutations, these lesions burst out of the duct or lobule into the surrounding fat and tissue. One mutated cell can reproduce and develop into an invasive tumor with its own blood supply. These cells may also spread through the lymphatic system or bloodstream to affect other organs. When this happens, the cancer is said to have *metastasized*. Breast cancer can spread to the bone, for example, and the cancer there would be considered and treated as metastasized breast cancer rather than bone cancer. The only way to stop this series of events is to stop the carcinogens, and the only way achieve that is to understand what they are.

Key Risk Factors: Leading the list of risk factors for breast cancer are exposure to toxic environmental estrogens called *xenoestrogens* (pronounced "zeno"-estrogens) and the use of the hormone estrogen. Environmental estrogens are dangerous for several reasons: they act like estrogen in the body; they cause our own estrogen to convert to cancer-causing forms of estrogen; they increase our risk of breast, ovarian and endometrial cancer; they promote infertility by suppressing progesterone; and they cause early puberty (*See* Ovarian Cysts, Precocious Puberty). Xenoestrogens are found in soft plastic products, plastic wrap, medical plastics used in IV bags and oxygen tubing, pesticide-laden foods (fruits, vegetables, dairy and meat), dioxins, cosmetics containing parabens, chemicals used to bleach feminine hygiene products, dry cleaning chemicals and nail polish. Dark hair dyes contain phenylenediamine, an estrogen-mimicker and known cancer-causing agent.

A study published in the *Journal of Applied Toxicology* in 2004 found that parabens were found in 18 of 20 breast tumors. Parabens are used extensively in cosmetics, pharmaceuticals and deodorants. Women who used anti-perspirants or deodorants, who shaved frequently and who started these habits before age 16, were found, in a study published in the *European Journal of Cancer Prevention*, to be diagnosed with cancer up to 22 years earlier than those who rarely used the products.

The hormone estrogen is commonly prescribed for Hormone Replacement Therapy (HRT) either alone or in combination with progestins. In July 2002, the debate about the safety of estrogen plus progestins finally ended: a Women's Health Initiative (WHI) study was halted when researchers noted an increased risk of blood clots, breast cancer, coronary heart disease and stroke in participants. In fact, the study group had a 26 percent increase in the risk of invasive breast cancer. This wasn't the first study to show a link between hormone therapy and breast cancer, but it is the one that caught the attention of the scientific community. As a result, the U.S. Food and Drug Administration finally listed estrogen as a carcinogenic agent. The FDA now recommends that hormone replacement therapy be used at the lowest doses and for the shortest period of time that will produce desired results.

Prolonged use of oral contraceptives is another controversial subject. Try natural fertility monitors to determine your fertility cycle and when you are at risk of becoming pregnant (go to www.hormonehelp and click on alternatives to the PILL). As well, be aware that some anti-depressants, cholesterol-reducing drugs and anti-hypertension medications increase the risk of breast cancer. Statins, used to lower cholesterol, also deplete the body of the breast protective nutrient coenzyme Q10 (Co-Q10). Silicone breast implants, especially those encased in polyurethane foam, cause trauma to breast tissue during implantation.

Early onset of menstruation, often the result of excess estrogen caused by xenoe-strogens, is also an issue, as is late onset of menopause. (*See* Precocious Puberty, Menopause) Being overweight or obese increases estrogen stores in fat, and can also contribute to breast cancer. (*See* Weight Management)

Poor diet also plays a starring role in the development of breast cancer, and is a factor in 35 percent of cases. Diets high in hormone containing meats, animal fats and dairy products are associated with breast cancer, as are cigarette smoking and the early or excessive consumption of alcohol. As fiber helps to pull excess estrogen from the body, diets that are low in fiber can be a factor in high levels of circulating estrogens, which promote breast disease.

PRESCRIPTION FOR HEALTHY BREASTS

Nutrient	Dosage	Action
Multivitamin with minerals: (FemmEssentials or MultiEssentials for women)	As directed. For complete formula recommendations see Appendix A.	Ensures adequate nutrient status
Milk Thistle	100 mg daily	Supports liver health, which is important for metabolism of hormones
Calcium D-glucarate	300 mg daily	Important for healthy metabolism of estrogen; detoxifies breast cancer-promoting agents
Turmeric (95% curcumin)	100 mg daily	Prevents breast cancer, detoxifies cancer-causing form of estrogen, excellent to reduce chemotherapy side effects
Indole-3-carbinol (found in cruciferous vegetables)	300 mg daily	Reduces risk of breast cancer, can be used in conjunction with tamoxifen;

		prevents healthy estrogen from converting into the cancer-causing form
Chaste Tree (Vitex) berry	100 to 175 mg daily	Balances estrogen-to-progesterone ratio
Evening Primrose oil	Six 500 mg capsules per day	Anti-inflammatory; controls negative prostaglandins involved in pain and inflammation
Green tea extract	200 mg daily	Protects against breast cancer
Rosemary extract	50 mg daily	Reduces tumor formation and breast lumps; antioxidant
Lycopene	10 mg daily	Antioxidant, reduces risk of breast cancer
Sulforaphane (found in from cruciferous vegetables)	400 mcg daily	Reduces risk of breast cancer

HEALTH TIPS TO ENHANCE HEALING

- Eat organic foods, especially organic dairy products, to avoid xenoestrogens. Focus on a diet high in organic vegetables, especially those from the cruciferous family: broccoli, cauliflower, kale and Brussels sprouts as they are high in the cancer fighter Indole-3 carbinol. Reduce your intake of sugar as it suppresses the immune system. Ensure that the fats you eat are those that are rich in essential fatty acids.

- Lignans are a plant estrogen found in very high concentration in flax seeds. Researchers at the University of Toronto believe that daily consumption of the lignans in flax seeds (which you can grind and sprinkle on your cereal every day) can help to prevent and treat breast cancer. Alpha-linolenic acid from flax seed oil has also been shown to have a breast cancer protective effect.

- Avoid nail polishes that contain formaldehyde or tolulene. Look for those that are phthalate-free. (pronounced *thay-late*) These xenoestrogens have been linked with reproductive disorders. Avoid dark hair dyes, which have been linked with cancer. Go blonde, or go natural! Safe, toxin-free products are available at your local health products store. Look for Herbatint in the health food store; it is a great natural hair dye.

- Use natural cosmetics that do not contain parabens. Find natural, toxin-free products at your health products store.
- Take EstroSense breast-supporting nutrients every day. *See* www.estrosense.com
- Protect your breasts from breast traumas as they promote DNA damage. Remember the more breast X-rays you have, the more DNA damage your cells will experience.
- Avoid clothes that need to be dry-cleaned, and use only unbleached sanitary products (NatraCare feminine hygiene products).
- Support new mothers to breastfeed as long as possible, as nursing is a potent protector against breast cancer.
- Avoid hormone replacement therapy; the combination of estrogen and progestin has been found to increase the risk of invasive breast cancer. Use herbal alternatives to treat menopausal symptoms (*see* Menopause).
- Exercise for a minimum of 30 minutes three times per week to reduce your breast cancer risk dramatically.

Candida albicans, see Vaginal Yeast Infection.

Cervical Dysplasia

The American College of Pathology states that four out of five women who die of cervical cancer had not had a PAP smear in the previous five years. According to Health Canada, the highest incidence of cervical cancer and the highest death rates occur in women over the age of 65, a group that often stops having annual PAP tests. PAP smears save lives by discovering abnormal cells, called cervical dysplasia, early enough to prevent loss of life from cervical cancer. Every adult woman from the age of 18 should have an annual PAP test to ensure her cervix is healthy—but what can be done when the test comes back abnormal? (*See* Appendix C for more information on PAP tests)

Symptoms
There are no symptoms until invasive cervical cancer makes itself apparent. This is why an annual PAP test is necessary.

Causes

We know the main risk factors that promote abnormal cervical cells include: greater number of sexual partners, increasing age, infection with the Human Papilloma Virus (HPV) (the virus that also causes warts), smoking, oral contraceptive use and nutritional deficiencies of folic acid, vitamin A and vitamin C.

We definitely do not want to ignore abnormal PAP tests. Too many women are advised they have an abnormal test result, told to come back in six months for another test and are not given any suggestions for how to get their cervical cells to return to normal. Yes, some abnormal cells return to normal with no treatment, but what if simply taking a nutritional supplement containing vitamin A and C and folic acid could ensure a normal PAP? Every woman I know would take a multivitamin with minerals to help those cells revert to healthy cells.

We know that HPV is implicated in the majority of cervical dysplasia and cervical cancer cases. New research has shown that a nutrient called Indole-3-carbinol can reverse abnormal cervical lesions before they have a chance to develop into cancer. In one study 30 women with CINII and CINIII cervical lesions took 200 mg or 400 mg of I3C daily. Fifty percent in the treatment group had complete regression of their lesions. None of the placebo group had complete regression of their lesions. Indole-3-carbinol is available in a nutritional supplement called EstroSense in the dosages used in the study to reverse abnormal cells. EstroSense also contains other nutrients, including calciumD-glucarate, rosemary containing carnosic acid, Milk thistle, lycopene, sulforaphane, tumeric and green tea—all researched to help prevent female cancers and keep our estrogens from converting to cancer-causing estrogens. So you get the benefit of returning abnormal PAP tests to normal while helping to prevent female cancers.

PRESCRIPTION FOR HEALTH

Nutrient	Dosage	Action
Multivitamin with minerals, (FemmEssentials or MultiEssentials for women)	As directed. See Appendix A for complete formula recommendations	Ensures adequate nutrient status

Milk Thistle	100 mg daily	Supports liver health, which is important for metabolism of hormones
Calcium D-glucarate	300 mg daily	Important for healthy metabolism of estrogen; supports normal cell growth
Turmeric (95% curcumin)	100 mg daily	Prevents abnormal cell growth, detoxifies cancer-causing form of estrogen
Indole-3-carbinol (found in cruciferous vegetables)	300 mg daily	Stops healthy estrogen from converting into the cancer-causing form. Has been shown to reverse abnormal PAP tests within 3 menstrual cycles
Chaste Tree (Vitex) berry	100-175 mg daily	Balances estrogen-to-progesterone ratio important for proper cell function
Evening Primrose oil	Six 500 mg capsules per day	Anti-inflammatory; controls negative prostaglandins involved in pain and inflammation
Green tea extract	200 mg daily	Protects against abnormal cell growth; detoxifies excess estrogens
Rosemary extract	50 mg daily	Reduces tumor formation; is antioxidant
Lycopene	10 mg daily	Antioxidant; reduces risk of cancer
Sulforaphane (found in cruciferous vegetables)	400 mcg daily	Reduces risk of cancer; stops abnormal cell growth

Constipation

Most alternative doctors have stopped asking their patients if they are regular because they always say "yes"–regardless if they have a bowel movement once a day or once a week. North Americans spend almost one billion dollars per year on laxatives. Each of us has been constipated at one time or another but 20 percent of us are chronically constipated. Few discuss the problem and what little knowledge that is gained usually comes from advertisements and laxative packaging.

Constipation occurs when it becomes necessary to strain in order to remove hard feces or when waste is not eliminated from the body in an appropriate amount of time. You should have at least one large bowel movement a day, or two to three smaller ones (about 12 inches of waste should be excreted in total). The feces should be soft, bulky and easy to pass.

Symptoms
Infrequent, small, hard and dry bowel movements that are difficult to pass are the main symptom. Constipation often results in hemorrhoids, skin problems, headaches, body odor and fatigue as well as irritability, depression, obesity, insomnia and diverticulitis. Waste that is left in the colon too long causes toxin build-up and can lead to more serious bowel disease and cancer.

Causes
When disease is not present, constipation usually arises when we don't drink enough water or eat enough fiber, eat too much protein and highly processed food or when we don't make enough time to have a bowel movement. A change in routine, business travel and restaurant eating can all promote constipation. The typical Western diet does not include enough whole, natural food and relies far too much on what is convenient, either fast foods or store-bought packaged foods that are processed to ensure a long shelf life and are devoid of fiber. Packaged food is also high in sugar, sodium, artificial flavors and chemical colorants that lead to constipation.

Other factors that can contribute to constipation are a lack of exercise, prolonged use of laxatives or antacids, nutritional deficiency, pregnancy, parasitic infection and yeast overgrowth. Constipation is also seen in people with low thyroid function, food allergies, or who take prescription medications or iron supplements.

PRESCRIPTION FOR HEALTH

Nutrients	Dosage	Action
Vitamin C	Take vitamin C to bowel tolerance, meaning start taking powdered C in gram doses mixed in juice or water every hour until lose stools occur; then cut back until stool is no longer loose. Then, as a preventative, take 500 mg twice daily.	Softens stools, promotes elimination and strengthens intestinal capillaries
Multivitamin with minerals (FemmEssentials or MultiEssentials)	As directed; see Appendix A for complete list of suggested nutrients	Aids metabolism, improves digestion
Magnesium citrate	Up to 1000 mg taken in divided doses throughout the day until stools are softened	aids elimination
Flax seed Oil & Omega's High Lignan Flax seed	1 to 2 tablespoons of the oil and powder daily. Make sure to drink water when taking ground flax seed	Soothes intestinal lining and promotes elimination
BB536 Bifidobacterium longum	2 capsules daily containing at least 5 billion live bacteria	Improves intestinal flora and reduces harmful bacteria
Artichoke	160 to 320 mg three times daily with meals, assuming standardized to contain 13-18% caffeolquinic acids calculated as chlorogenic acid	Increases bile formation and flow to digest and absorb fats

Cascara sagrada	Tea or capsules containing 250 mg for several days. Do not use continually	Improves peristaltic action of the colon
Pantothenic Acid	250 mg daily	Improves peristaltic action of the colon

HEALTH TIPS TO ENHANCE HEALING

- Take time each day to have a bowel movement. Preferably the same time every day. Do not be rushed, eventually the body will respond at the same time each day.
- Drink water—8 to 10 glasses of pure, filtered water a day, but do not drink during meals or else you will dilute your digestive enzymes. For every juice, alcoholic or caffeine beverage that you drink, add another 8 to 10 ounces. A study in Italy found that drinking 8 glasses of water daily, along with a high-fiber diet was more beneficial than eating a high-fiber diet alone.
- Do not use commercial laxatives because they promote dependence and chronic constipation. High-fiber foods such as prunes or other dried fruit, whole grains or seeds (especially ground flax seed or psyllium seed), and sauerkraut (or sauerkraut juice) are far more effective in alleviating constipation and support the body's functions naturally. (I like FiberLean, available in Canada by Brad King.)
- Eat vegetables or fruits at every meal; you want 7 to 10 half-cup servings per day. If you haven't been eating raw veggies regularly, start with steamed; they are easier on the digestive system. And remember—if your food comes from a box, it's bad for your bowels.
- Get plenty of exercise. Yoga or t'ai chi are great for improving circulation, reducing tension and promoting healthy digestion and elimination. Stretching exercises where you must touch your toes or draw your knees up to your chest are also good to get the bowels moving.
- Avoid deep-fried foods, food that is high in sugar and other refined carbohydrates (like white bread), caffeine, alcohol and dairy (except yogurt).
- If you suspect you have low stomach acid, take one capsule (600 mg) of hydrochloric acid before a large meal. If symptoms worsen, stop—you do not have low stomach acid. If you feel the same or better, increase your dosage by one at your next meal. Keep increasing dosage up to a maximum of seven capsules or until you feel warmth in your stomach. If you feel the warmth, cut

back your dosage prior to the feeling. Use fewer capsules for smaller meals.

Other Recommendations
- Get tested for food allergies or low thyroid function.
- When eating, ensure that the atmosphere is relaxed and pleasant. Don't work through lunch or dinners, or eat hunched over the coffee table or standing over the sink. The benefits of spending 15 to 20 minutes sitting and enjoying your meal far outweigh the time saved eating on the run.
- For quick relief, magnesium oxide taken before bedtime will flush out your system the next morning. It turns stools to liquid and cleans trapped waste out of the small pockets in the intestines.
- If you need to take additional iron, try a liquid iron supplement like Floradix; it is non-constipating.

Health Fact

Before you say, "It's just easier to use a laxative," consider this: not only do over-the-counter laxatives not address the problem of why you are constipated, they actually make the problem worse. Regular use of laxatives disturbs the body's natural rhythm. In essence the body forgets how it is supposed to eliminate waste. Also, laxatives are drugs that can cause nutritional deficiencies. The unnatural increase in gut motility can prevent calcium and vitamin D absorption. Some products can prevent the absorption of fat-soluble vitamins and folic acid.

Diabetes

Diabetes is a serious condition affecting 6.3 percent of the population according to the American Diabetes Association. The World Health Organization (WHO) predicts that 300 million people worldwide will have diabetes by the year 2025. Those are alarming figures, particularly since the disease is preventable with simple lifestyle changes. Complications of diabetes include blindness, erectile dysfunction, kidney disease, gangrene and heart disease. According to the Canadian Diabetes Association, 80 percent of those with diabetes will die from heart disease or stroke.

There are three forms of diabetes. Type 1 diabetes is also known as Insulin Dependent Diabetes Mellitus (IDDM) or juvenile diabetes; it typically strikes before the age of 30. It occurs when the pancreas no longer produces sufficient insulin, a crucial hormone in the transportation of sugar to our cells. In over 85 percent of those with Type 1 diabetes, the immune system destroys the pancreatic insulin-secreting beta cells. The inability of the pancreas to produce insulin causes glucose to build up in the bloodstream. Because glucose is not transferred to the cells, the cells starve.

Type 2 diabetes, also called Non-Insulin Dependent Diabetes Mellitus or NIDDM affects about 90 percent of those diagnosed with diabetes. Those with Type 2 diabetes tend to be overweight and over 40, but increasingly today we are seeing more Type 2 diabetes in young children. In Type 2 diabetes, although the pancreas may produce low or normal amounts of insulin, the peripheral organs and tissues have become resistant to insulin's effects.

Gestational diabetes occurs in about two to five percent of pregnancies. Those who develop gestational diabetes and their offspring are at much higher risk of diabetes later in life.

Symptoms
Symptoms of diabetes include excessive hunger and thirst, frequent and copious urination, and weight fluctuations: Type 1 generally causes weight loss, and Type 2 is associated with weight gain. Watch for cuts and bruises that are slow to heal, and tingling or numbness in your hands and feet. Extreme lack of energy, itchy skin and blurred vision are also involved. Recurring bladder and vaginal yeast infections may also be present. Skin tags that grow on the neck, face, armpit, groin and the folds under the breasts are also a sign of diabetes. Sixty percent of those with skin tags have diabetes. Type 2 diabetes is an insidious condition, with symptoms appearing so gradually that they often go unnoticed.

Causes
Type 1 diabetes results from damage to the cells in the pancreas responsible for insulin production as a result of a virus, infection or other immune system destruction. It is also possible that an allergy to the albumin in milk promotes destruction of the insulin-producing cells. Mothers are encouraged to breast-feed their children, as clinical research shows that breastfed infants do not develop Type 1 diabetes as often as those on milk-based formulas. Researchers

have found that the introduction of gluten-containing foods before the age of six months may also increase the risk of developing Type 1 diabetes in children.

A growing body of research has found a connection between diet and lifestyle and the development of Type 2 diabetes. The Western diet of high sugar and high fat, coupled with a lack of fruits, vegetables and fiber leaves many people undernourished and overweight. Insulin is the main hormone that contributes to our weight problem. The standard, high-carbohydrate, low-protein diet is disrupting our bodies' ability to regulate blood sugar adequately. When we are pumping out too much insulin to reduce abnormally high blood glucose, we inevitably gain weight and become fat, and our cells become resistant to insulin and weight loss. Everyone who is overweight has insulin resistance, and this resistance puts them at a higher risk for diabetes as well as cancer and heart disease. Those with an apple-shape or "beer belly," with excess weight around the middle, are at serious risk of disease. In North America, one in four children between the ages of two and five are obese. Over 60 percent of the adult population is overweight, and 15-30 percent are considered obese.

PRESCRIPTION FOR HEALTH

Nutrient	Dosage	Action
Multivitamin with minerals (FemmEssentials or MultiEssentials)	As directed. See Appendix A for complete nutrient recommendations	For complete nutrient support
Vitamin C (buffered with mineral ascorbates)	1000-2000 mg per day in divided doses	Prevents vitamin C deficiency and reduces Sorbitol and aldose reductase (an enzyme that causes many diabetic complications). High Sorbitol can damage sensitive tissues in the eyes causing retinopathies. Vitamin C protects against retinopathy.

Alpha Lipoic Acid	100-200 mg three times daily	Converts glucose to energy, protects against free radical damage, improves insulin sensitivity, recycles vitamin C and stops neuropathies
Chromium picolinate	100-200 mcg three times daily	Improves blood sugar levels, stimulates the synthesis of fatty acids and cholesterol. Lowers triglycerides and cholesterol. Improves insulin sensitivity
Holy Basil	100-200 mg three times per day	Lowers blood sugar, reduces total cholesterol, decreases cortisol. Regulates blood pressure by reducing the effects of stress
Bilberry Extract	20-40 mg three times daily. Dosages of 600 mg per day for diabetics with retinopathy	Improves retinopathy and strengthens capillaries
Gymnema sylvestre	75-150 mg three times per day of standardized to 75% Gymnemic acids daily	Research studies in humans showed it lowers blood glucose, and increases insulin; a reduction in medication was required and no side effects were reported. A rat study found an increase in the number of islet and beta cells of the pancreas and the pancreas increased in weight by 30 percent.
Fenugreek extract	1000 mg daily	Lowers blood sugar levels and improves insulin sensitivity. Normalizes cholesterol.

Bitter Melon	Either fresh, unripe bitter melon or 100-200 mg three times per day in capsules	Has a similar affect as insulin. Normalizes blood glucose
Milk thistle	600 mg per day standardized to 80 percent silymarin	Protects the liver, a potent antioxidant; protects the pancreas from toxicity. Silybinin, a component of silymarin, improves insulin sensitivity while inhibiting glucose-stimulated insulin release. Reduces insulin requirements
Nopal cactus	50-100 mg three times per day	Mild effect in lowering blood glucose and total cholesterol. Use in combination formulas with other glucose-regulating herbs.
PGX	As directed	Suppresses appetite, stabilizes blood sugar. It reduced after-meal blood sugar by 20 to 40 percent and insulin secretion by about 40 percent, reducing a whole body insulin sensitivity index by 50 percent. PGX lowers the glycemic index of the meal consumed.
Omega-6 Fatty acids – Evening Primrose or Borage Oil	4000 mg of Evening Primrose oil or 2000 mg of Borage oil per day	Improves diabetes-related peripheral nerve dysfunction and increases the enzyme activity on Omega-6 that is inhibited by abnormal blood glucose and insulin levels.

Omega-3 Fatty Acid	Pharmaceutical grade fish oil providing 600 mg of both EPA and DHA	Lowers blood pressure, increases levels of good cholesterol, reduces the level of bad cholesterol and lowers the levels of fibrinogen, a protein that makes blood thicker and stickier. Also necessary for the formation of prostaglandins.
Flax seed Fiber	1 to 2 tablespoons of ground flax seed	Slows the absorption of carbohydrates. Decreases total cholesterol and triglycerides and blood sugar levels.

HEALTH TIPS TO ENHANCE HEALING

- Research published in the *Journal of Epidemiology* 2002 found that by taking a vitamin and mineral supplement, the risk of developing diabetes was reduced by 30 percent in men and a 16 percent in women. Basic nutrients are the foundation on which you will build your personalized anti-diabetes program.

- Eat small, frequent meals high in protein. Dietary changes are a priority for those with diabetes. Adopt the simple rule of not eating any white foods– white sugar, white flour, white pasta, white rice, white potatoes, etc. Eat brightly colored fruits and vegetables because they are high in vitamins and minerals and low on the glycemic index. Regular consumption of fruits and vegetables reduces the risk of developing diabetes. The Finnish Diabetes Prevention Study Group found that lifestyle modifications using diet and exercise reduced the incidence of diabetes in high-risk men and women by almost 60 percent.

- Avoid all processed foods. Processed foods (containing sugars and trans-fatty acids) and refined carbohydrates take only a few minutes to cause a rapid increase in blood sugar and corresponding release of insulin. A complex or non-refined carbohydrate can take hours to convert to glucose. Hence the reason this book recommends "good carbohydrates" only. Research published in the *American Journal of Clinical Nutrition* states that women eating a diet high in trans-fatty acids have an increased risk of developing diabetes.

- In addition to avoiding white foods, attention should be paid to the level of dietary fiber in the diet. Up to 40 grams of fiber should be eaten daily by those with diabetes.

- To increase your intake of EPA and DHA, add regular servings of fish such as salmon, herring or mackerel. Eat only good fats and eliminate trans-fatty acids from your diet (found in processed foods). When saturated fats (the bad ones) are replaced with essential fats from flax, fish, borage, evening primrose, olive oil, avocados, nuts and seeds, insulin levels normalize or decrease.

- Eliminate artificial sweeteners (aspartame, Sweet'N Low, sucralose) and use stevia (containing no sugars and having zero calories). Stevia has been shown to have a positive effect on the pancreas. Xylitol (which has been researched to prevent periodontal disease) is another sweetening option for those with diabetes.

- Avoid alcohol and cigarettes. Alcohol is high in sugars. Cigarette smoking increases insulin resistance and high circulating blood insulin levels.

- Eat small amounts of protein throughout the day. Protein, when eaten in small amounts, inhibits the rise of glucose and stimulates glucagon to release stored carbohydrates in the liver. But too much protein has been shown to increase insulin, especially when consumed with certain types of carbohydrates. When simple, refined carbohydrates are combined with too much protein—for example, the burger with the white bun—insulin increases. Consume good protein sources with excellent carbohydrate sources low on the glycemic index, while adding good fats and avoiding sugars.

- Avoid or greatly reduce processed meats such as hot dogs and bologna. Aside from increasing your cancer risk, research has shown that eating processed meats five or more times per week is a risk factor for developing diabetes.

- Walking as little as 30 minutes per day can dramatically reduce the side effects associated with diabetes while aiding the return of normal blood glucose and insulin regulation. Losing as little as 2-14 percent of excess body fat has been shown to reduce triglycerides, high cholesterol, normalize fasting blood glucose and plasma insulin.

- Have your doctor check for hypothyroidism or do the Barnes Basal Body Temperature Test in Appendix C to determine if you have functional hypothyroidism.

Endometriosis

The Endometriosis Association states it is extremely rare that a woman in this day and age should ever need a hysterectomy for endometriosis, no matter how severe. Yet, three out of four gynecologists I visited said, "You have already had your children, so if we find that you have extensive endometriosis during laparoscopy, the best option is to perform a hysterectomy." This was in response to yet undiagnosed severe pelvic pain. The thought of a hysterectomy sent me searching for the cause for the intense pain I was experiencing. All my symptoms seemed to point to endometriosis. Finally, the fourth doctor I visited discussed diagnosis and treatment options with me without mentioning hysterectomy as a "cure." That was over a decade ago and today I am still free of endometriosis (and doctors are still recommending hysterectomies).

Symptoms

Endometriosis is one of the most common yet misunderstood female diseases. Approximately 15 percent of women between the ages of 20 and 45 years of age are affected with this painful and debilitating disorder. Symptoms can begin with the onset of menstruation and progressively increase with pending menopause. Dysmenorrhea (pain with menses), dyspareunia (pain with intercourse), and infertility may also be present. The pain some women experience can be devastating. Pain worse than childbirth was my only symptom and, strangely, the pain radiated from my left hip into my back. Many women also experience pain when they have a full bladder or bowel. Some women experience no pain but may have fertility, ovarian or menstrual problems. The symptoms are many and vary from woman to woman.

Careful Diagnosis: Pelvic examinations by a highly skilled gynecologist may disclose nodules or lesions on the ovaries. Ultrasound tests will only show endometriosis if the ovaries are involved. Laparoscopy is the only diagnostic technique that can clearly determine if endometriosis is present. This examination, performed under general anesthetic, involves inserting a light-containing telescope through a small incision in your navel and another one or two small incisions along the bikini line for the instruments.

A laparoscopy is only as good as the surgeon who performs the exam. Removing all the endometriosis tissue requires a physician who is committed to biopsy and getting rid of all suspicious abnormalities. My surgeon was meticulous and I was rid of endometriosis in one surgery.

Endometrial tissue can look like tiny blueberries or black spots; white, yellow or reddish cysts, varying from tiny bluish or dark brown blisters to large chocolate cysts up to 20 centimeters in diameter. Only biopsy can confirm which tissue is truly endometriosis.

It is not uncommon for endometrial cells to grow on the ovaries, the fallopian tubes, the pelvic ligaments, the outer surface of the uterus, bladder, the large intestine and the covering of the abdominal cavity. Women are often misdiagnosed with irritable bowel syndrome, bladder infections, appendix attack, "just" PMS or painful cramps.

Causes

Until recently, the most predominant theory to explain the cause of endometriosis was that of retrograde menstrual flow. It was believed that blood flowing backward pushed tiny fragments of normal endometrial tissue (from the lining of the uterus) up the fallopian tubes where it took up residence in the abdominal or pelvic cavity. Here this tissue acted as it would in the uterus in accordance with the monthly menstrual cycle. The blood often could not escape, however, and caused the formation of deposits and severe pain.

Other researchers believe that retrograde menstruation occurs, but it is only in those women with altered immune function that the endometrial tissue implants on other body areas. In other words, your immune system should not allow the endometrial tissue to survive where it does not belong. Once this abnormal tissue is present, the immune system may mount an antibody response and create inflammation and pain in the region involved.

New research points to a glitch in the immune system. Dr David Redwine, world renowned expert and director of the Endometriosis Program at St. Charles Medical Center in Bend, Oregon, believes that some women are born with abnormally located endometrial cells and that something goes awry with the immune system, causing the cells to become active. This theory has gained acceptance because endometrial implants have been found in the nose, lungs and organs far from the uterus. Dr. Redwine has a website where further information on his technique can be found www.empnet.com/scmc/redwine.html or phone 541-383-6904.

Environmental Pollutants Linked to Endometriosis: Convincing evidence has linked organochlorine exposure to the development of endometriosis. Organochlorines are persistent, toxic substances, like DDT, PCP and dioxins. They are estrogen mimickers, causing an increase in estrogens in the body. Endometriosis is thought to be higher in women who have higher than normal circulating estrogens. Carolyn De Marco, in her book *Take Charge of Your Body*, states that dioxins are a group of 75 chemicals used to make PVC plastics (our drinking water runs through pipes made from PVC in our homes), solvents, pesticides, refrigerants and in the pulp and paper industry. These same chemicals also persist in the fats of meat and dairy products. The EPA estimates that 90 percent of human dioxin exposure is through food, primarily meat and dairy products.

Endometriosis is an insidious disorder but it can be cured forever if you examine and reduce your stress levels, reduce the environmental toxins you are exposed to and improve your nutrition. I eliminated my endometriosis for good, and you can too.

Seven Early Warning Symptoms of Endometriosis

1. Menstrual cramps that increase in severity
2. Intermenstrual pain, usually at mid-month
3. Painful intercourse or dyspareunia
4. Infertility of unknown origin
5. You think you have bladder infection, but the test results are negative
6. Pelvic pain that is all-encompassing
7. History of ovarian cysts

PRESCRIPTION FOR HEALTH

Nutrient	Dosage	Action
Multivitamin with minerals; *no iron* FemmEssentials or MultiEssentials for women	As directed. See Appendix A for complete information.	Ensures adequate nutrient status

Milk Thistle	100 mg daily	Supports liver health, which is important for metabolism of hormones
Calcium D-glucarate	300 mg daily	Important for healthy metabolism of estrogen; supports normal cell growth
Turmeric (95% curcumin)	100 mg daily	Prevents abnormal cell growth, detoxifies cancer-causing form of estrogen
Indole-3-carbinol (found in cruciferous vegetables)	300 mg daily	Stops healthy estrogen from converting into the cancer-causing form. Has been shown to reverse abnormal PAP tests within 3 menstrual cycles
Chaste Tree (Vitex) berry	100-175 mg daily	Balances estrogen-to-progesterone ratio; important for proper cell function
Evening Primrose oil	3000 mg per day	Anti-inflammatory; controls negative prostaglandins involved in pain and inflammation
Green tea extract	200 mg daily	Protects against abnormal cell growth, detoxifies excess estrogens
Rosemary extract	50 mg daily	Reduces tumor formation; antioxidant
Lycopene	10 mg daily	Antioxidant; reduces risk of cancer
Sulforaphane (found in cruciferous vegetables)	400 mcg daily	Reduces risk of cancer; stops abnormal cell growth

Natural progesterone cream	In Canada, progesterone cream is a prescription drug. Use 6% natural progesterone 1/4 to 1/2 tsp morning and night between day 5-28 (or whenever your normal cycle ends). In the U.S., ProgestaCare by Life Flo is niceas it delivers 20 mg in a pre-measured pump dose.	Limits the endometrial tissue build-up caused by estrogen
Cramp Bark tincture	1/2 teaspoon every 2-4 hours for acute pain	Relaxes the uterus and reduces cramps

HEALTH TIPS TO ENHANCE HEALING

- Take EstroSense containing Indole-3-carbinol, d-glucarate, sulforaphone, green tea, curcumin, milk thistle, rosemary and lycopene.
- The key to eliminating endo is NO dairy products. Dairy products promote the prostaglandins and leukotrienes that cause inflammation, cramps and pain. Dairy also contains xenestrogens.
- Excess estrogens must be eliminated. Reduce your consumption of estrogens from pesticide-laden foods; buy organic foods whenever possible.
- Reduce stress in your life. Working women with type-A personalities are the most prone to endo. Women who are constantly under stress from their job, family pressures and personal expectations are at higher risk for developing endometriosis. In Tori Hudson's book *The Women's Encyclopedia of Natural Medicine*, she states that, "Baboons who developed endometriosis in captivity were found to have higher stress levels and a decreased ability to react to stress compared to those in the wild," suggesting stress is a factor.
- Get regular exercise to ensure that circulation in the pelvic area is restored. If you sit all day, your lower abdomen becomes congested.
- A special endometriosis tea formula was developed by herbalist Rosemary Slick. A healthy liver is essential for hormonal regulation because it converts active ovarian estrogen (estradiol) into the safer form (estriol). She recommends that women with endometriosis drink three to four cups of this tea per day for four to six months.

> **Endo-Tea**
>
> 3 parts dandelion root
>
> 3 parts wild yam root
>
> 2 parts burdock root
>
> 2 parts pau d'arco bark
>
> 1 part vitex berries
>
> 1 part Oregon grape root
>
> 1/2 parts dong quai root
>
> Sassafras, cinnamon, orange peel and ginger to taste
>
> • *Combine herbs. Fill a large pot with four cups of cold water. Add four to six tablespoons of the herb mixture. Simmer over low heat for 20 minutes. Strain.*

Other Recommendations

- Refuse to use bleached paper products containing dioxins (estrogen mimickers) —this includes toilet paper, sanitary napkins and especially tampons.
- Do not use plastic containers to store food or water they contain estrogen mimickers. Do not microwave in plastic as the estrogens leach into the food.

Pain Relief: Castor oil packs are excellent at controlling pain. Take six pieces of flannel soaked in castor oil (damp but not dripping) about the size of the area you want to treat. Cover these flannel pieces with a hot water bottle wrapped in a towel and place on the lower abdomen for 30 to 45 minutes, several times a day. This will not only relieve pain but also improves circulation in the pelvic area.

Drug Side Effects: Because of the hormone connection, medical therapy for endometriosis has concentrated on altering a woman's hormonal chemistry with drugs. These drugs include Danazol, gonadotropin-releasing hormones (GnRH) such as Nafarelin and birth control pills.

Drugs can be successful in alleviating endometrial symptoms, but not without side effects. They include acne, breast reduction, depression, oily skin, appearance of facial hair and weight gain. Some may induce menopausal symptoms such as lowered libido, vaginal dryness, hot flashes and a loss in bone density. No drug can cure the disease. Upon withdrawal, the endometriosis symptoms return. Holistic treatment that allows the body to heal itself is more effective and much safer.

Fibromyalgia

Almost 16 million North Americans suffer from fibromyalgia (FM), a multi-system disorder and common rheumatic syndrome that has also been referred to as the "invisible illness" because of the difficulty in diagnosing it. The name fibromyalgia is rooted in Latin: *fibro*, meaning supportive tissue; *myo*, for muscle; and *algia* for pain. The hallmark of fibromyalgia is widespread pain throughout the muscles, stiffness and chronic aching. It affects women more than men, and usually strikes between the ages of 30 and 60 years. It accounts for 15 to 30 percent of all visits to rheumatologists.

The pain of FM is thought to be caused by a tightening and thickening of the thin film of tissue that holds muscles together. A diagnosis of FM will be confirmed if your doctor finds pain or tenderness in 11 out of 18 trigger points located in the knees, hips, rib cage, shoulder and neck.

Many of the symptoms of FM overlap with those of chronic fatigue syndrome (CFS). The main symptom difference between the two is profound fatigue in CFS and muscle pain in FM. Treatments for chronic fatigue syndrome focus on the elimination of viruses that may be causing the fatigue whereas FM treatments look at reducing the inflammatory factors that cause the pain and swelling of joints and muscles. Due to the many symptoms of FM and chronic fatigue, a combination of therapies may be required to get the conditions under control.

Symptoms

The symptoms of FM are varied and no two sufferers are the same. They can include: allergies; anxiety; mental confusion; fatigue; dysmenorrhea; ridged fingernails, stiffness; inability to exercise; gastrointestinal problems; depression; mood swings; headaches; irritation by light, sound or odors; dizziness; anxiety; mental confusion; heart palpitations; sleep disturbances; carpal tunnel syndrome; skin is tender to the touch; swollen joints; total body aches and pain. Non-restorative sleep is a major symptom where those affected sleep but never feel rested.

When people describe their muscle fatigue, they liken it to shoveling snow or gardening for days without a break, or that the muscles are being stretched and torn.

The unique nature of the each person's collection of symptoms makes FM difficult to diagnose. Many tests including urine, blood, CAT scan, magnetic resonance imaging, X-ray and more may be conducted without any clear indication of what is wrong with the person, and often sufferers are referred to psychiatrists. Life becomes unbearable for those living with FM. It can also be difficult for family and friends to understand this shadowy disease.

Causes

No one cause can be pinpointed but it is believed that multiple stressors, a traumatic emotional or physical event and depressive episodes that upset the functioning of the immune system contribute to the disorder. It is suspected that a connection lies between FM and chronic fatigue syndrome as those with FM usually have a history of extreme, relentless fatigue. Viruses may have a hand in it, such as Epstein-Barr virus or fungus like *Candida albicans*. New research is showing that undetected Lyme disease may be the root cause. Heavy metal and chemical toxicity, as well as nutritional deficiencies, are major players in the progression of FM. Allergies are also thought to play a role in FM, and they must be diagnosed and eliminated to allow healing. Low serotonin levels and low DHEA are also seen in those with FM. Physicians must peel away the causal layers of each symptom and treat each symptom individually in order to eliminate this disorder.

The Inflammation Factor: The immune cytokine Interleukin-6 is one factor responsible for causing pain and inflammation. High levels of the stress hormone cortisol cause the immune system to secrete inflammatory factors and high cortisol also causes DHEA levels to drop. FM sufferers generally have very low DHEA levels. DHEA is an important anti-inflammatory hormone, reducing pain symptoms effectively. Many FM sufferers have found that none of the supplements they try work. There is a good reason for this. FM is made worse by the release of interleukin-6 and unless we turn off this powerful inflammatory immune factor we are not getting to the root of the problem.

PRESCRIPTION FOR HEALTH

Nutrient	Dosage	Action
Multivitamin with minerals (FemmEssentials or MultiEssentials)	As directed; *see* Appendix A for complete list of suggested nutrients.	Aids metabolism, improves digestion
Celadrin, both oral and topical	1500 mg per day Topical apply twice per day	Anti-inflammatory, reduces pain and swelling of joints
Magnesium (either or a combination of any of the following forms: citrate, fumarate, glycinate, malate, succinate or aspartate)	200 mg three times daily	Needed for 300 enzymatic reactions; calms muscles
Malic Acid	1200-2000 mg daily	Detoxifies the body of aluminum and reduces pain of FM. Works synergistically with magnesium
5-HTP	50-100 mg three times per day	Increases serotonin levels, reduces anxiety, muscle pain, improves sleep and early morning stiffness; enhances mood; controls appetite
St. John's wort, standardized hypericin	100-300 mg three times per day	Effective for depression and enhances serotonin levels. Do not take with prescription anti-depressants without medical supervision
Valerian	As directed	Improves sleep, calms nerves

DHEA	5 mg per day	Helps to normalize cortisol levels
Melatonin	1-3 mg per night	Improves sleep
L-carnitine	500 mg daily	Improves energy production and eliminates fatigue

HEALTH TIPS TO ENHANCE HEALING

- Eat a balanced diet of fresh fruit and vegetables, healthy oils, nuts and seeds, whole grains and fresh wild fish to fight FM. Eat smaller meals more frequently throughout the day to maintain blood sugar levels.
- Avoid processed, refined foods; they are high in sugar, salt and hydrogenated fat.
- Drink plenty of pure, filtered water—8 to 10 glasses daily. For every beverage (other than herbal tea) that you consume, drink another glass of water.
- Eliminate alcohol, smoking and caffeine.
- Get regular exercise, but don't overexert yourself. Gentle, moderate exercise improves your circulation and enhances your mood and overall well-being. Even walking to your mailbox or sitting in a chair and raising your arms and legs can be beneficial.

Other Recommendations

- Laugh! Rent videos, see a stand-up comic and hang around funny friends. Laughter as well as exercise can improve mood. Keep a positive frame of mind.
- Ensure adequate rest.
- Practise deep breathing exercises to ensure sufficient oxygen intake.
- Detoxification is extremely important. Saunas allow toxins to excrete from the skin; dry brushing before a shower or bath will increase circulation and stimulate lymph flow; and internal herbal cleanses combined with fiber will eliminate waste from the intestines and support the liver and kidneys. Have an Epsom salts and baking soda bath every night. Pour one cup of each into a bath; run the water through your shower filter rather than the tap to ensure you are not soaking in chlorinated water.
- Start a diet diary and write down everything you eat and see if there is any increase in symptoms or their intensity after eating certain foods. Ask for a referral to an allergy specialist and get tested for possible triggers. Once you

know what you are allergic to, avoid those allergens. Environmental allergies should be tested as well.

- Have dental amalgams removed to reduce your toxic load.
- Massage, acupuncture and chiropractic treatments can help speed healing.
- When you are having a bad day, rest. On your good days, enjoy them to their fullest without overexerting yourself.
- Since there are multiple causes to this illness, there are multiple cures. What works for one person may not work for another due to biochemical individuality. Do not give; the most important gift is the power of faith.

Fibrocystic Breast Disease

With the fear of breast cancer so prominent today, breast lumps are a concern for many women. Fibrocystic breast disease (FBD), also called *cystic mastitis*, is a common, non-cancerous condition. It can be mildly uncomfortable to severely painful, especially when breasts become swollen. Fluid that has not been drained via the lymphatic system fills in small spaces within the breast. The fluid is then encapsulated by fibrous tissue and thickens like scar tissue. The cysts may swell before and during menstruation. Although it does not increase your risk of cancer, it may make detecting cancerous tumors difficult through breast self-exams.

Twenty to 40 percent of women who are pre-menopausal (between the ages of 35 and 50) experience FBD, with the symptoms generally disappearing after menopause. FBD is affected by the rise and fall of monthly female hormones.

Symptoms
Breasts are a mixture of fat, glands and connective tissue so their texture will always be irregular. Breast tissues are affected by a woman's monthly hormonal cycle. During the cycle, milk-secreting glands enlarge with fluid and their cells multiply. Most of the excess fluid is reabsorbed or drained by the lymphatic system. This occurs month after month and year after year. In some women this process causes fibrous tissue to develop into lumps. Symptoms include breast tenderness and swelling, and a lumpy feeling to the breast.

It can be very distressing to feel these lumps. Monthly breast self-exams, infrared breast scans and/or ultrasound can help lay your fears of breast cancer to rest. If a breast lump is discovered, have your physician assess it and don't worry–most lumps are benign. Lumps that suddenly grow larger and don't change with your menstrual cycle; discharge from your nipple; severe, unrelenting pain or puckered or dimpled skin on your breast should be reported to your physician immediately. (*See* Breast Self-exam in Appendix C)

Causes

FBD occurs when there is excess estrogen or an imbalance in estrogen to progesterone in the body due to stress, estrogen replacement therapy or due to xenoestrogens. It is also seen in young women with irregular periods. Lumps may come and go, with symptoms often disappearing after menstruation has passed and hormone levels return to normal. Because of its timing, it is considered a symptom of PMS. It is now considered a risk factor for or precursor to breast cancer.

Heavy coffee consumption has been linked to FBD, along with a diet high in "bad" fats. As well, being overweight is a risk factor for FBD.

PRESCRIPTION FOR HEALTH

Nutrient	Dosage	Action
Multivitamin with minerals; *no iron* FemmEssentials or MultiEssentials for women	As directed *See* Appendix A for complete nutrient recommendations	Ensures adequate nutrient status
Milk Thistle	100 mg daily	Supports liver health, which is important for metabolism of hormones
Calcium D-glucarate	300 mg daily	Important for healthy metabolism of estrogen; supports normal cell growth

Turmeric (95% curcumin)	100 mg daily	Prevents abnormal cell growth, detoxifies cancer-causing form of estrogen
Indole-3-carbinol (found in cruciferous vegetables)	300 mg daily	Stops healthy estrogen from converting into the cancer-causing form. Has been shown to reverse abnormal PAP tests within 3 menstrual cycles
Chaste Tree (Vitex) berry	100 to 175 mg daily	Balances estrogen-to-progesterone ratio; important for proper cell function
Evening Primrose oil	Six 500 mg capsules per day	Anti-inflammatory; controls negative prostaglandins involved in pain and inflammation
Green tea extract	200 mg daily	Protects against abnormal cell growth, detoxifies excess estrogens
Rosemary extract	50 mg daily	Reduces tumor formation; antioxidant
Lycopene	10 mg daily	Antioxidant; reduces risk of cancer
Sulforaphane (found in cruciferous vegetables)	400 mcg daily	Reduces risk of cancer; stops abnormal cell growth
Potassium Iodine or kelp	As directed	Important for thyroid activity. Deficiency of iodine promotes FBD symptoms. See Thyroid
Evening Primrose oil	3000 mg per day	Anti-inflammatory; controls negative prostaglandins involved in pain and inflammation

Natural Progesterone cream	20 mg from day 5 to 28, or until period begins	Restores progesterone level and alleviates estrogen dominant symptoms

HEALTH TIPS TO ENHANCE HEALING

- To reduce estrogen levels, follow an organic, predominantly vegetarian diet and increase your fiber intake. Fiber carries estrogen out of the body.
- Detoxification and elimination of waste is very important. Eat liver-friendly foods such as lemons, onions, garlic, leeks, kale, carrots, beets, artichokes and members of the cabbage family (broccoli, Brussels sprouts, cauliflower).
- Avoid caffeine, chocolate, tea and cola drinks as they contain methylxanthines that cause FBS.
- Treat constipation to ensure elimination of toxins (*See* Constipation).
- Take EstroSense containing Indole-3-carbinol, d-glucarate, sulforaphone, green tea, curcumin, milk thistle, rosemary and lycopene.

Other Recommendations

- Exercise regularly to improve circulation, and help to detoxify and manage weight.
- Rule out low thyroid. See Appendix C for a home thyroid test.
- Do self-exams monthly to familiarize yourself with your breasts so that you are able to detect subtle changes such as thickening, lumps, etc., and when they occur or disappear.
- Avoid antiperspirants, they clog up drainage from the sweat glands and the toxins have to drain back into the breast. Also they contain parabens which are linked to breast cancer.
- Massaging your breasts in a circular motion will improve lymph flow and circulation, while at the same time familiarizing you with their architecture. Make it a daily ritual, either during your morning shower or before you go to bed.
- To control pain, use castor oil packs. (*See* Endometriosis for how-to information.)

Heart Disease

Heart disease is the number one killer of women of all ages each year. We have finally achieved equality as women now have equal rates of heart disease to men, although more women are dying of heart attacks than men are. Nearly one out of two women will die of cardiovascular disease. Women are also more likely than men to suffer a stroke after a heart attack. We have been taught that a heart attack is signalled by arm-clutching chest pain, but women can have very different heart attack symptoms to men. Unfortunately, many women are not aware that the risk is so great and do very little to protect themselves from the disease. Cardiovascular disease is a category of about 30 conditions including hardening of the arteries, congestive heart failure, heartbeat rhythm irregularities, heart muscle disease and valve disorders.

Symptoms

Heart disease is a silent killer because often people do not know that they have it. New statistics published by the American Heart Association (AHA) for 2004 show that 50 percent of men and 64 percent of women who died suddenly of heart disease during the course of their study had no previous symptoms. Be conscious of heart disease symptoms, including shortness of breath, irregular heartbeat, chest pain with exercise that subsides when you rest, or bouts of indigestion, a constricting feeling in your throat, profuse sweating for no apparent reason (not menopause). Seek emergency help for stomach pain, nausea and vomiting, dizziness, irregular pulse, light-headedness or unusual fatigue, and pain or numbness in the arms, back, neck or chest.

Causes

Although you may be predisposed to heart disease because of family history, this does not mean you must develop it. If you have a family history of coronary heart disease (CHD) you must be vigilant in making lifestyle choices that can prevent this deadly condition. Heart disease actually begins in the stomach. A poor diet of packaged or processed foods high in trans-fatty acids and devoid of fiber and nutrients (especially B vitamins and folic acid) are the main instigators of heart disease. Couple a poor diet with high stress, dehydration, aging, smoking, extra weight and lack of exercise and sleep and your risk climbs higher. Diabetes, high blood pressure or high levels of harmful LDL cholesterol or high blood homocysteine levels compound the problem. Homocysteine in the blood indicates a breakdown in chemical processes in the body, and is strongly linked to heart disease. The risk of CHD is especially high for women of African-American descent.

PRESCRIPTION FOR HEART HEALTH

Nutrient	Dosage	Action
Multivitamin with minerals, *no iron* (FemmEssentials or MultiEssentials)	As directed. See Appendix A for complete formula recommendations	Ensures adequate intake of basic nutrients. For the prevention of heart disease B vitamins (normalizes homocysteine, reduces stress), folic acid, magnesium, vitamins C and E are essential
Magnesium	300 mg daily	Alleviates arrythmias, heart palpitations; essential for proper heart muscle function
Vitamin B1 for those taking Lasix	60 mg daily	To prevent B1 depletion in those taking Lasix
Vitamin C with bioflavonoids	1000 mg twice a day; with bioflavonoids 100 mg per day	Reduces symptoms and risk of heart disease; anti-oxidant, which raises HDL "good" cholesterol and lowers blood pressure
Potassium	500 mg per day	Maintains healthy blood pressure
Coenzyme Q10	100 to 300 mg daily	Boosts energy production in the heart muscle; significantly improves heart function in those with congestive heart failure

Inositol hexanicotinate Nonflushing niacin	500-1000 mg three times per day with meals. If using just niacin, increase dosage slowly over three weeks until using 3000 mg per day to avoid the harmless flushing of the skin	Lowers LDL cholesterol and triglycerides while raising HDL cholesterol. Have liver enzymes and cholesterol checked every three months
Vitamin E with mixed tocopherols	200-400 IU daily	Improves blood flow, reduces fatty plaques, boosts the immune system and acts as an antioxidant. Should not be taken by those on Warfarin
Hawthorn extract (standardized 1.8% vitexin or 10% procyanidin content)	100-200 mg three times daily	Double-blind studies show improvement in those with congestive heart failure
Coleus forskohlii	5-10 mg per day	relaxes arteries, reduces blood pressure
Garlic	2000-4000 mg of Kyolic garlic	Improves circulation, shown to reduce blood pressure
Pycnogenol or grape seed extract	100 mg twice daily	Reduces platelet aggregation
Gugulipid (standardized extract of mukul myrrh tree)	500 mg three times daily (standardized for 25 mg guggulsterone)	Increases the liver's metabolism of LDL cholesterol, lowers LDL cholesterol and triglyceride levels and raises HDL cholesterol levels; also shown to prevent atherosclerosis and reverse pre-existing plaque
Omega-3 fatty acids	Pharmaceutical grade fish oil, 400 mg EPA and 200 mg DHA daily	Reduces risk of heart disease; lowers triglycerides

HEALTH TIPS TO ENHANCE HEALING

- Studies show that a diet emphasizing fresh fruits and vegetables, whole grains, legumes, lean meats and fish may lower risk of heart disease. Eating this way also provides valuable antioxidants, which are useful in combating chronic inflammation. Eat two eight-inch raw carrots per day, as this has been shown to reduce cholesterol by 50 points in a matter of weeks. Eat plenty of fresh pressed garlic to lower blood pressure.

- The AHA recommends two servings of fish per week to prevent heart disease. Fatty fish contains EPA and DHA, Omega-3 essential fatty acids. Alternatively, be sure to supplement with essential fatty acids to lower triglyceride levels and support normal cardiovascular health.

- Make sure that you keep hydrated with adequate amounts of pure, filtered water to maintain blood flow. Studies show drinking 5 glasses of water per day cuts your risk of stroke and heart attack in half.

- Reduce consumption of salt, caffeine and alcohol and be sure to get plenty of exercise followed by sufficient rest.

- Have your thyroid checked. Low levels of thyroid hormone causes heart palpitations in women and adds to heart stress.

- Quit smoking and avoid second-hand smoke.

- Insist that your doctor measure your homocysteine and C-reactive protein levels (both indicators of heart disease). Fortunately, high levels can be quickly addressed by supplementing magnesium, B6, B12, folic acid and fish oils.

- Studies show that holding on to anger is not only bad for your mood, but is also linked to increased risk of heart disease.

- A common culprit found in people with high blood pressure is the wrong ratio of potassium to salt. Reduce sodium intake by avoiding table salt and processed foods. Increase your intake of potassium-rich foods such as bananas, apricots, tomatoes, avocados, potatoes, lean chicken meat and fresh fish.

- Get adequate exercise. Walking 30 minutes three times a week cuts your risk of heart attack by about 30 percent. The more energetic your exercise, the greater your benefit: increasing your walking pace to two miles per hour or faster can reduce your risk up to 63 percent.

Caution: If you are currently on Coumadin, high cholesterol or high blood pressure medication, talk to your physician or pharmacist about drug-nutrient interactions. Be aware that both high blood pressure and high cholesterol medications cause depletion of coenzyme Q10 so you must supplement to ensure adequate levels. According to the *Drug-Induced Nutrient Depletion Handbook for Pharmacists*, if you are taking Lasix (flurosemide) you should be aware that Lasix depletes calcium, magnesium, potassium, vitamins B1, B6 and C and zinc. These nutrients must be replaced to prevent deficiency.

Menopause

Menopause means one year with no menstrual period. Peri-menopause is the 10 to 15 years before menopause and everything after the periods have stopped for one year is post menopause. The average age of menopause is 52 years. At menopause the ovaries have stopped producing eggs and there is no possibility of pregnancy. Smoking, medication, surgery (oophorectomy), radiation and autoimmune disease that affects the ovaries can trigger premature menopause. Menopause is not a disease, but rather is a natural milestone in every woman's life.

Symptoms

On average, 70-80 percent of women will experience mild to moderate symptoms, while 10-15 percent will suffer with severe symptoms and may require hospitalization. The most obvious symptom is the cessation of menses. Symptoms include anxiety, hot flashes and night sweats, problems with sleep, vaginal itching (with or without discharge) brain fog, memory problems, mood swings, irritability, depression, migraine headaches, new environmental allergies and food sensitivities, weight gain, urinary incontinence (aggravated by coughing, sneezing or laughing), recurring urinary tract or vaginal infections. Increased risk of heart disease and bone loss are also associated with menopause in susceptible women. *See* Osteoporosis and Heart Disease for more information on how to prevent and treat these serious conditions.

Causes

Menopause is a natural phase in a woman's life. When our ovaries stop producing estrogen, our adrenal glands are supposed to kick in and provide us with the estrogen we need. Our fat cells also produce estrogen and so does the uterus. Then our liver processes and packages those hormones and the thyroid hormones play a role. What makes the difference between a woman who has no symptoms at menopause and the woman who suffers with a multitude of the symptoms mentioned above? Women with exhausted adrenals, low levels of thyroid hormones and a congested liver will have terrible menopause symptoms compared to women with a healthy liver, thyroid and adrenals. (*See* Adrenal Exhaustion and Thyroid for more information.) Low levels of thyroid hormones cause extreme hot flashes and night sweats, vaginal dryness and flooding, irregular periods. Exhausted adrenals promote insomnia whereby you go to bed and fall asleep just fine, but wake up three hours later and are unable to return to sleep.

Most women have been taught they are estrogen deficient, yet we are overloaded with toxic environmental estrogens that contribute to our hormonal problems and increase our risk of breast and ovarian cancer at menopause. (*See* Breast Cancer for more information on xenoestrogens)

HRT Concerns: Hormone Replacement Therapy (HRT) has hit its demographic sweet spot—with the largest number of baby boomers turning 45 in 2004, expected sales will be in the multi-billions. HRT was originally developed to halt the symptoms of menopause, but doctors also prescribed HRT to prevent cardiovascular disease and bone loss, keep teenage girls from growing too tall, relieve depression, reduce urinary incontinence, stop colon cancer and Alzheimer's disease and to keep us young forever. It became the panacea for all sorts of women's conditions and was touted as the "fountain of youth" even though the safety of HRT was still being heavily debated. No randomized, controlled clinical trials were ever conducted to verify that HRT should be used for all those conditions, and its safety in healthy women was never proven. In July 2002, the Women's Health Initiative study, a clinical trial designed to determine if HRT was beneficial to healthy women, was halted five years and two months into the study due to serious safety concerns. This study, which was supposed to last eight years, involved 16,608 healthy, postmenopausal women (meaning they had stopped their periods for 12 months), who were at low risk for heart disease. The women received 0.625mg of equine (horse) estrogen (Premarin) along with 2.5 mg of synthetic progestins for 5.2 years. Premarin (made by Wyeth-Ayerst) contains estradiol plus at least two or more horse estrogens, such as equilin and equilenin. The study concluded that the combination of estrogen and progestins posed a significant health risk to women and that any benefits from HRT were not worth the side effects. The study found a 41 percent increase in the risk of stroke, a 29 percent increase in the risk of heart attack, a doubled risk of blood clots, a 22 percent increase in cardiovascular disease and a 26 percent increase in the risk of invasive breast cancer.

Later in 2003, scientists reported that women who took the combination of estrogen and progestins also developed such dense breast tissue that it was extremely difficult to detect breast cancer on a mammogram. Those women also had higher rates of adult-onset asthma. Worse yet, women taking these hormones were found to have double the risk of developing dementia. But the estrogen-only arm of the WHI study was still allowed to continue until 2004, when they halted it due to increased risk of stroke, dementia and mild brain damage. Hopefully, women will pay attention to these results and avoid HRT. Less than 10 percent of all menopausal women will need some type of hormones for extreme, uncontrollable hot flashes and night sweats; the rest can use natural herbs, vitamins, minerals and lifestyle changes.

PRESCRIPTION FOR MENOPAUSE SYMPTOMS

Nutrient	Dosage	Action
Multivitamins with minerals (FemmEssentials or MultiEssentials)	As directed. See Appendix A for complete nutrient formula	Supports optimal nutrient status
Vitamin C with bioflavonoids (particularly hesperidin)	600 mg per day, 100 mg citrus bioflavonoids	Decreases the number of hot flashes; hesperidin, a bioflavonoid, also reduces night leg cramps
Vitamin B6 (pyridoxal-5-phosphate or pyridoxine)	50 mg daily vitamin B6 along with a B-complex daily	Supports nervous system, required for metabolism and immune function, reduces PMS symptoms

Vitamin E (d-alpha tocoperhol with mixed tocoperols)	200-400 IU daily	Reduces hot flashes and improves mood. If needed, use vaginal lubricants containing natural vitamin E (d-alpha, not dl-alpha).
Calcium with magnesium	1000 mg calcium; 250-500 mg magnesium daily	Reduces leg cramps and restless legs, helps prevent constipation, osteoporosis, supports proper cardiovascular function
Indole-3-carbinol	150-300 mg daily	Eliminates excess toxic and cancer-causing estrogens
Ginkgo biloba (standardized to 24%)	40 mg three times per day	Supports cognitive function; improves circulation to hands and feet
Chaste tree (Vitex)	80-160 mg one to two times daily	Supports proper hormone secretion; reduces PMS symptoms; controls hot flashes.
Dong Quai (only in combination formulas with other herbs including Black cohosh)	100-200 mg one to two times daily	Balances estrogen activity; tones uterus; reduces spasms; beneficial for cardiovascular system
Black cohosh (1 mg of triterpene glycosides measured as 27-deoxyacteine)	80-160 mg one to two times daily. If you have night sweats take 160 mg at bedtime	Reduces depression, insomnia, vaginal dryness and hot flashes; nonestrogenic, found safe for those with estrogen-receptor positive breast cancer
Hesperidin	75-150 mg one to two times daily	Stops hot flashes and night sweats; stops night leg cramps

Gamma oryzanol (from rice bran oil)	75-150 mg one to two times daily	Relieves hot flashes; supports pituitary function and promotes endorphin release by the hypothalamus, thereby improving mood. Lowers triglycerides and total cholesterol
5-HTP	50-100 mg three times per day	Increases serotonin levels; reduces anxiety, muscle pain; improves sleep and early morning stiffness. Enhances mood; controls appetite
Melatonin	1-3 mg per night	Improves sleep
Omega-3 Fatty Acids	1000 mg three times per day	Relieves breast pain; may alleviate hot flashes
St. John's wort	100 mg twice daily	Alleviates depression. Do not take in addition to antidepressant medications without first consulting your doctor

HEALTH TIPS TO ENHANCE HEALING

- Eat a diet rich in cruciferous vegetables (broccoli, Brussels sprouts, cauliflower, cabbage and kale). You should have at least two half-cup servings per day. Cruciferous vegetables contain Indole-3-carbinol and sulforaphane, important nutrients for maintaining balanced hormones in our liver while reducing our risk of breast cancer. Add flax seeds, fennel, chickpeas, lentils and soy to your diet for their hormone-balancing action.

- Walk briskly and swing your arms. Walking briskly every day for 30 minutes cuts hot flashes by 50 percent, while improving your heart and bone health at the same time. If you are having trouble sleeping, take 100 mg of 5HTP three times a day (breakfast, dinner and before bed) to improve your mood and aid restful sleep.

- Take Black Cohosh, Dong Quai, Vitex, Gamma oryzanol and hesperidin found in MenoSense to reduce night sweats, hot flashes, vaginal dryness, heavy erratic periods, mood swings, weight gain and sleep disturbances. Your health food store carries a variety of menopause formulas containing different combinations of these herbs. Take a multivitamin with minerals every day along with essential fatty acids and bone-building nutrients to ensure your heart and bones are protected.

- Eat breakfast every day. Over 40 percent of women do not eat breakfast. Research has shown that women who skip breakfast are at higher risk of heart disease than those who eat bacon and eggs for breakfast often. Eating a protein-rich breakfast ensures that you have adequate amino acids to make the mood-enhancing and sleep-inducing serotonin.

- Reduce the stress in your life. Have a massage at least once a month. Start looking after yourself. Do one thing you love to do at least once a day. Tell your loved ones you "need" extra love, attention and help. It is OK to ask.

- Address any underlying thyroid and adrenal imbalance or gut dysbiosis like *Candida albicans* and be sure to cleanse and support the function of the liver and colon.

- Ask your doctor for a dual energy X-ray absorptiometry (DEXA) scan to check your bone density. DEXA is the gold standard for determining osteoporosis.

- Enjoy sexual intercourse twice a week to prevent vaginal atrophy and to maintain high levels of immune function.

- Look at menopause as a beginning rather than an end. Try things that you have always wanted to do but had no time for when you were raising young children and building your career.

- Read my book, coauthored with Dr. Karen Jensen, ND, called *No More HRT: Menopause Treat the Cause* for in-depth information on menopause.

Menstrual Abnormalities

A normal menstrual cycle involves complex hormonal interactions that stimulate the ovaries to produce and release estrogen, progesterone and ova (eggs). Menstruation normally occurs in the first five days of the cycle as a result of a decline in estrogen and progesterone levels when pregnancy does not occur. Without these hormones to support the uterine lining, it pulls away, tearing capillaries and causing bleeding.

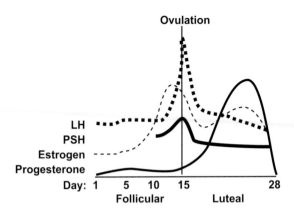

In the follicular phase (Days 6-14), a shift in follicle-stimulating hormone and luteinizing hormone (LH) triggers production of estrogen from the ovaries, which encourages the growth of a new uterine lining, known as the endometrium. At the midpoint of the cycle, rising estrogen levels cause LH levels to surge, and in response, the ovaries release an egg, typically between Days 12 and 14.

In the next phase, Days 14 to 28, the site of egg release (corpus luteum) secretes copious amounts of progesterone, necessary to prepare the endometrial lining to receive a fertilized egg. At this stage in the luteal phase of the cycle, progesterone levels exceed estrogen levels. If pregnancy does not occur, progesterone and estrogen levels drop, leading to menstruation, and the cycle begins again.

Cycles continue until an average age of 52 years and would normally only be interrupted by pregnancy and breastfeeding. Hormonal problems, including imbalances in the estrogen/progesterone ratio, can interfere with normal cycles. Problems with menstruation include amenorrhea (absent periods), menorrhagia (excessive bleeding), dysmenorrhea (extremely painful menstruation) and irregular periods. There is often a variety of underlying conditions that prompt these symptoms.

Amenorrhea

Amenorrhea means the absence of periods. Periods typically begin in the early teens, and should continue, unless pregnancy occurs, until menopause. A physician should examine girls who haven't started puberty by age thirteen, or who start puberty but do not menstruate within five years, and girls who have reached the age of sixteen without menstruating.

Amenorrhea may be caused by an abnormality in the pituitary gland, brain, adrenal glands, ovaries or other components of the reproductive system. Thyroid imbalances are often a factor in infrequent or lack of periods (*See* Thyroid). Hormonal irregularities such as polycystic ovary syndrome may prevent the release of an egg, disrupting the hormonal cycle. (*See* Polycystic Ovary Syndrome) High levels of stress or Cushing's syndrome can cause the production of excess cortisol, suppressing production of the necessary reproductive hormone DHEA, and resulting in the disruption of periods. Anorexia, excess exercise and being overly thin may interfere with the menstrual cycle, as can scarring of the uterus or placental tumors called *hydatidiform moles*.

Menorrhagia

Menorrhagia means heavy bleeding. Approximately 75 percent of abnormally heavy bleeding is the result of hormonal imbalances that interfere with the proper functioning of the reproductive system. Sustained high levels of estrogen are typically involved. Hydatidiform moles, uterine fibroids and polycystic ovary syndrome may also be present. (*See* Uterine Fibroids, Polycystic Ovary Syndrome). Low levels of thyroid hormone are also a cause of heavy bleeding (*See* Thyroid).

Physical causes of heavy bleeding include adenomyosis (abnormal growth of uterine cells), which is often found in girls whose mothers took diethylstilbestrol (DES). These girls are at increased risk of vaginal and cervical cancer when they are older. Injury from sexual abuse, infection or prolapse of the uterus can also cause bleeding. The National Hemophelia Association predicts that up to three percent of women suffer from undiagnosed bleeding disorders such as von Willebrand disease, a genetic disease caused by a deficiency or a defect of a crucial blood clotting protein. Deficiency in Vitamin K, vital for blood clotting, may also be a factor in heavy bleeding. Excessive blood loss can lead to anemia (*See* Anemia).

Dysmenorrhea

Dysmenorrhea is marked by painful cramps, headache, nausea, vomiting and frequent urination, with menstruation severe enough to interfere with the normal activities of 5 to 15 percent of women. Primary menstrual pain may result from uterine contractions that occur when blood supply to the endometrial lining diminishes. The expulsion of clots is also a source of pain. Secondary dysmenorrhea can be the result of such conditions as endometriosis, adenomyosis (abnormal cell growth), fibroids and abdominal adhesions. (*See* Uterine Fibroids, Endometriosis)

Whether you are experiencing heavy periods, painful periods or no periods, these abnormalities must be reported to your doctor. Be sure that you receive a referral to a gynecologist, who should perform an ultrasound (either vaginal or abdominal) to help discover the cause of your symptoms. Abnormal bleeding, pelvic pain or abdominal fullness should not be ignored.

PRESCRIPTION FOR HEALTH

Nutrient	Dosage	Action
Multivitamin with minerals, *no iron* FemmEssentials or MultiEssentials for women	As directed See Appendix A for complete nutrient recommendations	Ensures adequate nutrient status. Vitamin B6, magnesium are essential for treating menstrual abnormalities
Milk Thistle	50 mg daily	Supports liver health, which is important for metabolism of hormones
Calcium D-glucarate	150 mg daily	Important for healthy metabolism of estrogen; supports normal cell growth; combined with I3C and sulphoraphane, stops abnormal periods and period pain
Turmeric (95% curcumin)	50 mg daily	Prevents abnormal cell growth, detoxifies cancer-causing form of estrogen

Indole-3-carbinol (found in cruciferous vegetables)	150 mg daily	Eliminates excess toxic and cancer-causing estrogens. Has been shown to reverse abnormal PAP tests within 3 menstrual cycles. Halts flooding periods and normalizes menstrual cycle.
Chaste Tree (Vitex) berry	100 to 175 mg daily	Balances estrogen-to-progesterone ratio. Normalizes menstrual cycle and stops PMS.
Evening Primrose or Borage Oil	3000 mg per day of Evening Primrose oil or 2000 mg of Borage oil daily	Anti-inflammatory; controls inflammatory prostaglandins involved in pain and inflammation. Stops diarrhea and flooding periods.
Green tea extract	100 mg daily	Protects against abnormal cell growth; detoxifies excess estrogens
Rosemary extract	25 mg daily	Reduces tumor formation, is antioxidant
Lycopene	5 mg daily	Antioxidant, reduces risk of cancer
Sulforaphane (found in from cruciferous vegetables)	400 mcg daily	Reduces risk of cancer. Stops abnormal cell growth. Halts flooding periods and abnormal menstrual cycle.
Cramp bark tincture	2 to 8 mL of root tincture	For spasmodic dysmenorrhea
Potassium Iodine or kelp	Follow directions on the label	Important for thyroid activity. Deficiency of iodine promotes heavy periods and infertility.

| Natural Progesterone cream | 20 mg from day 5 to 28 days or until period begins | Restores progesterone level and alleviates estrogen dominant symptoms. Controls heavy bleeding. Also used to promote menstruation. |

HEALTH TIPS TO ENHANCE HEALING
See Endometriosis for health tips.

Osteoporosis

Our bones are in a constant state of regeneration as bone is being broken down and rebuilt. Hormones, our liver, kidneys and immune system all work together to ensure that bone is maintained. Osteoporosis, meaning "porous bone," arises when bone is broken down faster than it can be rebuilt. Over time a gradual decrease in bone mass causes the bones to become porous, brittle and fragile, increasing the risk of fracture. Bones of the hip, spine, wrists and ribs are the most common fracture sites. Osteoporosis affects almost 30 million people, over 80 percent of those are women. One in four women has osteoporosis and one in eight men. Hip fracture is a dangerous result of osteoporosis. Over a quarter million hip fractures occur each year and over 50 percent will result in some form of disability, with many patients never getting out of long-term care facilities. Hip fractures result in death in up to 20 percent of cases.

If you have several of the risk factors mentioned below, have a dual-energy absorptiometry DEXA scan performed to determine bone status.

Major risk factors for osteoporosis

- Family history
- Low Stomach Acid
- Thyroid disease
- Corticosteroid therapy (prednisone)
- High-stress lifestyle or type A personality
- Northern European or Asian descent
- Thinness, small build
- Early menopause
- Sedentary lifestyle
- No pregnancies
- Smoking
- High caffeine and sugar intake
- High-protein diet

Symptoms

Bone loss occurs silently and often symptoms are not noted until a fracture occurs. Warning signs include: back pain around the bottom of the shoulder blades. The pain is relieved with heat, but aggravated by lying flat on the back. Teeth may become loose, there is a loss of height and a rounding of the upper back known as dowager's hump. Bones can fracture with little stress and collapsing vertebrae can pinch nerves, causing sciatica.

Causes

If we believe what the media have been telling us, we would think that calcium loss is the only cause of osteoporosis and that simply taking doses of calcium would solve the problem. Unfortunately this is not true—calcium alone will not reverse or halt bone loss in most suffering osteoporosis. Actually, studies using calcium alone have shown bone loss, not bone gain. Hormones, our immune system, stress and nutrition combine to maintain proper bone health.

Those with low stomach acid will have a difficult time absorbing calcium carbonate, the most common calcium used in supplements. Less than 10 percent of calcium carbonate is absorbed in those with low stomach acid. Calcium citrate, aspartate and orotate are much better absorbed. Calcium concentration is controlled by several hormones (including calcitonin secreted by the thyroid gland) and is influenced by our immune system.

Vitamin D also plays an important role in the formation of bone. Vitamin D interacts with the cells of the immune system by reducing the inflammatory cytokines, specifically interleukin-1 and interleukin-12. Carl Germano, RD and William Cabot, MD state in *The Osteoporosis Solution* that, "In some research circles, osteoporosis is thought to be a type of autoimmune disease."

The inflammatory cytokines of the immune system, specifically IL-1 and IL-6, can cause calcium to be pulled from bone. When we are under stress, our stress hormone cortisol is secreted. Cortisol release signals the T-helper-2 cells to secrete IL-6 and IL-6 . As well, when cortisol levels go up, our anti-aging and immune regulating hormone DHEA decreases. The body is designed to deal with short-term stressors, but when they become a regular occurrence, the cortisol/interleukin-1 and-6 connection causes a breakdown of bone faster than it can be rebuilt.

Osteoporosis can also be influenced by an overactive immune system. When macrophages eat invaders in the course of their daily surveillance, they release nitric oxide and IL-1. Nitric oxide in small amounts protects against bone loss. But when the immune system is fighting infection, macrophages release nitric oxide in large amounts, promoting the breakdown of bone. The drug Fosamax is designed to reduce nitric oxide, although with some terrible side effects. As mentioned earlier, we know that IL-1 also promotes bone loss so not only does vitamin D have to be available to control the secretion of IL-1, but our macrophages have to be kept in balance as well. Nitric oxide, like vitamin D, is key to regulating bone.

Estrogen protects the body from excessive secretion of IL-1 and IL-6. Lack of healthy estrogen in women with adrenal exhaustion or those who have had hysterectomies, or top-level athletes with suppressed menses, is associated with abnormally high levels of IL-1 (which promotes bone loss) and low levels of interferon gamma (which prevents bone loss).

The thyroid hormone thyroxin activates bone breakdown, so long-term elevated levels of the hormone for a prolonged period either through hyperthyroidism or too high a dose of medication for hypothyroidism also results in bone loss. Sub-clinical low thyroid function, where not enough thyroid hormone is available, also promotes bone loss.

Use of medications can also contribute to osteoporosis: corticosteroid drugs decrease absorption of calcium, and antidepressants have been linked to increased risk of hip fractures. Drugs such as diuretics, antacids, anticonvulsants, warfarin and lithium can also contribute to bone weakening.

Other factors promoting osteoporosis include genetic predisposition (Asians and Caucasians are at higher risk), hyperparathyroidism, hypothyroidism, excessive alcohol consumption, leanness, never being pregnant, side effects of prescription medication, immobility or lack of exercise and not getting enough sunlight. Smoking increases inflammatory immune factors promoting bone loss.

Calcium to Magnesium ratio: Research shows that the body requires twice as much calcium as magnesium. Taking more magnesium than calcium can actually suppress calcium levels and increase bone loss by decreasing the production of the thyroid hormone calcitonin. Magnesium in excess acts as a calcium blocker. There are times when we would want extra magnesium for restless leg syndrome, constipation, painful periods or heart palpitations, but we should then take the magnesium in divided doses at a different time than the calcium supplement.

PRESCRIPTION FOR BONE HEALTH

Nutrient	Dosage	Action
Multivitamin with minerals, *no iron* (FemmEssentials or MultiEssentials)	As directed. See Appendix A for complete formula	Ensures adequate nutrient status
Calcium chelate/ citrate/glycinate	1000 to 1500 mg, taken in divided doses with meals and/or at bedtime	Reduces bone loss; protects against fracture
Vitamin D	400 to 800 IU daily	Helps increase calcium absorption and inhibits IL-1 and IL-12 (known to promote calcium loss)
Vitamin K	150 mcg daily	Enhances osteocalcin, important for bone mineralization and increased bone strength

Magnesium (taken in a 2:1 ratio with calcium)	250-500 mg daily	Essential for absorption of vitamin D and to prevent deficiency
Boron (also found in broccoli powder)	3 mg to 5 mg daily	Reduces calcium excretion and mimics the beneficial effects of estrogen on bones
Quercetin	50-100 mg twice daily	Inhibits inflammatory response of IL-8, which promotes calcium loss
Turmeric (95% Curcumin)	25-100 mg daily	Inhibits inflammatory IL-1 and IL-6, known to promote calcium loss
Omega-3 Fatty Acids, pharmaceutical grade fish oils	1000 mg three times daily	Inhibits inflammatory IL-1, IL-6, and proinflammatory prostaglandins, known to promote calcium loss
Silicon (Biosil)	12 to 25 mg daily	Important for the formation of collagen in bone.
Ipriflavone	200 mg three times per day	Improves calcium absorption in bone, and slows osteoclast activity due to excessive nitric oxide; natural estrogen-like activity on bone only. Works better than prescription calcitonin. Combined with calcium enhances bone density considerably

HEALTH TIPS TO ENHANCE HEALING

- Look for bone supplements containing the majority of the nutrients mentioned above. We are waiting far too long to take our calcium supplements. Most women do not start taking calcium until age 50. Young women need calcium, especially during the crucial bone-building years 12 to 25.

- *See* Menopause. If you have osteoarthritis as well as osteoporosis *see* Arthritis.

- Rule out hydrocholoric acid deficiency. Low stomach acid impairs calcium absorption.

- Reduce consumption of caffeine (it depletes calcium and magnesium), simple or refined sugars (also depletes calcium and lowers bone density), and alcohol (it can lower vitamin D metabolism).

- Include more fermented soy in the diet from tempeh, miso, fermented soy powders and soy sauce.

- Eat plenty of green leafy vegetables; they contain vitamin K needed for proper bone mineralization.

- Eliminate all soft drinks; they lower calcium levels and increase phosphate levels.

- Reduce salt, it increases calcium loss.

- Maintain a balanced daily intake of protein—50 grams for women (average body weight of 138 lbs), 63 grams for men (average body weight of 174 lbs). Too much protein depletes calcium from the bones; too little prevents collagen formation and associated enzymes. Reduce animal protein by opting for vegetable-based protein such as legumes.

- Develop an adequate exercise program that includes weight-bearing activities such as walking, hiking, stair climbing, dancing, weight training, jogging, skiing or low-impact aerobics. However, while regular movement and exercise is required to preserve bone mass and increase bone mineral density, excessive exercising can also lead to osteoporosis if menses are suppressed or the immune system is hyper-stimulated.

- Eat calcium-rich foods including canned salmon with the bones, broccoli, sesame and sunflower seeds, dark leafy vegetables, organic cheese and yogurt. Take your calcium supplements before bed with a glass of orange juice. The blood's calcium level is lower at night so the rate of calcium absorption is greater.

- "Good fat" diets enhance bone density. High saturated fat diets promote bone loss.

- If your medication increases risk of osteoporosis, inquire if more natural approaches can be taken, or substitute it for one that does not. (Prednisone, Depo-Provera, steroids, blood thinners and diuretics are examples of drugs that increase risk.)

- Quit smoking.
- Take advantage of sunny days when you can and get at least 15 to 20 minutes of sunshine.
- Avoid antacids—they lower the acid in your gut and inhibit the absorption of calcium.
- Vitamin D is essential for the absorption of calcium into bone, and our bodies are capable of producing this vitamin when we are exposed to sunlight for about 20 minutes per day. You can see how this is a problem during the winter months. A Swiss study shows that supplementing vitamin D also helps to reduce the risk of falls for the elderly. Magnesium is essential to convert vitamin D to its active form and yet magnesium deficiency is common in the elderly population as well as in those with osteoporosis. Symptoms of magnesium deficiency include muscle cramps and twitching eyelids.
- Ipriflavone has been researched in over 60 different clinical studies, 16 of which are randomized, double-blind, placebo-controlled human studies. This compound is found naturally occurring in foods and plants. The richest source is alfalfa. It is also found in propolis from bees. Ipriflavone stimulates the synthesis and secretion of calcitonin from the thyroid gland. It also stimulates bone formation and increases bone density. It is more effective than prescription calcitonin at building bone and decreases fracture rates. Ipriflavone also inhibits inflammatory immune factors that pull calcium from bones. No bone rebuilding program should be without ipriflavone.

Ovarian Cysts, Polycystic Ovary Syndrome and Ovarian Cancer

Ovarian cysts

Ovarian cysts are very common and often exist without symptoms. In a normal cycle, every month several follicles, each containing an egg, develop. A surge of luteinizing hormone and follicle-stimulating hormone helps release the egg and progesterone increases. If the egg is not fertilized, the cycle starts all over again. Sometimes, however, no egg is released. Then no progesterone is secreted and more estrogen is released, thus maturing the follicles into fluid-filled sacs or cysts that will grow larger every month until progesterone is secreted.

Cysts can appear in a very short time and disappear just as quickly. Cysts can be alone or in groups, small or large (even as big as a lemon!). Often when cysts are a few centimeters in size, doctors will recommend surgery. However, if a diet and supplementation program is followed, those cysts will usually reduce and disappear. The risk of cancer increases when cysts become solid. Ovarian cancer is rare, but it is difficult to diagnose and remission rates with conventional medicine are poor.

Sometimes a follicle is able to grow tissue or skin cells within the cyst. These types of cysts will not dissipate and must be surgically removed.

Symptoms

Often ovarian cysts are not noticed until a pelvic examination is performed by the doctor or by an ultrasound scan. This is why it is so important to go for your annual PAP test because doctors perform a pelvic exam at the same time. For those with symptoms, the most obvious symptom is pain, either tenderness to the touch or a constant sore or burning sensation in the abdomen, located in the lower abdomen off to the right or left. Pain may occur during ovulation or intercourse. If a cyst erupts in the pelvic cavity, blood and fluid will discharge, possibly causing pain.

Causes

Ovarian cysts occur when there is a hormone imbalance. Estrogen dominance brought on by poor elimination of waste by the lymphatic system, colon, liver and kidneys is a factor. Emotional or physical trauma, prolonged stress, and even heavy exercise, can cause increased estrogen. A diet rich in meat and dairy products is also responsible for elevating estrogen. Cysts that occur after menopause should be looked at by a physician, as there is a greater risk of them being cancerous. The risk of ovarian cancer is increased with the use of fertility drugs or birth control pills, or if you have never been pregnant.

Polycystic Ovary Syndrome

Polycystic ovary syndrome (POS) is a disorder where many fluid-filled cysts are present and male hormones are excessively high. In this disorder, excess luteinizing hormone increases the production of male hormones that can cause acne and coarse hair growth.

Affecting up to ten percent of the U.S. population, Polycystic Ovary Syndrome is the most common hormone dysfunction among women in their reproductive years. Because eggs are frequently not released, fertility is a problem. If pregnancy does occur, it often ends with first trimester miscarriage or is associated with gestational diabetes. The condition seems to run in families, with 20 percent of mothers and 40 percent of sisters of those with PCOS also demonstrating varying degrees of the syndrome. With the approach of menopause, androgen production declines leading to a more normal pattern of menstruation. If left untreated, PCOS can lead to cancer of the uterine lining. Women with PCOS also are at increased risk for development of Type 2 diabetes, cardiovascular disease and hypertension.

Symptoms

PCOS usually shows with coarse hair growth on the face and chest, and higher levels of male androgenic hormones caused when the pituitary gland releases an excess of luteinizing hormone. Acne and oily skin are also evident. Ovaries are typically enlarged and contain multiple cysts. Symptoms often become apparent in puberty when menstruation is to begin: irregular menstrual periods with copious bleeding may occur, or PCOS can cause a lack of periods altogether. Infertility is a major concern of women with PCOS.

Causes

Although historically considered a gynecological problem, research now shows that PCOS is associated with hyperinsulinemia (production of too much of the insulin hormone) and impaired glucose metabolism. Perhaps not surprisingly, then, more than 65 percent of women who suffer from PCOS are obese. Reports indicate that early pubarche (breast budding and pubic hair growth) is linked to ovarian hyperandrogenism and insulin resistance, suggesting another hormonal trigger. Doctors typically try to determine if a tumor is responsible for the production of male hormones. Thyroid and prolactin abnormalities should also be investigated as possible causes of amenorrhea (lack of period).

Since the extra weight seems to be an important issue, those with PCOS should work toward losing excess weight gradually, using proper nutrition and exercise. Doing so will also lessen risks for diabetes and cardiovascular disease.

Ovarian Cancer

Ovarian cancer is the fifth most diagnosed cancer, accounting for almost five percent of all cancer deaths. In fact, about one in 70 women will eventually develop ovarian cancer. Known as the silent killer, vague symptoms make this cancer difficult to detect and allow it to invade other tissues. Ovarian cancer normally strikes between the ages of 50 and 70, and with an almost 60 percent death rate, women need to understand the symptoms so that they can seek treatment early.

Symptoms

Symptoms of ovarian cancer can mimic common illness and are often vague. According to the Canadian Cancer Society, symptoms of early stage ovarian cancer include a mild discomfort in the lower part of the abdomen, a sense of incomplete evacuation of stool, gas, a frequent need to urinate, indigestion, feeling full after a light meal, low back pain and vaginal discharge. More advanced symptoms include painful intercourse, abnormal bleeding, diarrhea or constipation, abdominal pain, nausea, vomiting and fatigue. A build-up of fluid in the abdomen makes clothes feel tight. At this point, a woman may lose weight or become anemic.

Tests to diagnose ovarian cancer are simple, and include a transvaginal ultrasound, a CA-125 blood test and a pelvic exam. Many doctors believe that the CA-125 blood test is not reliable, but the National Ovarian Cancer Association recommends it be done on women with above-noted symptoms. A 1983 Harvard University study found elevated levels in 80 percent of women with stages three and four ovarian cancer. The test was not as reliable with stage one and two cancer, and test results can also be high in women with uterine fibroids and endometriosis. Despite its imperfections, it is the best test that we have when combined with a transvaginal ultrasound. Fortunately, the CA-125 is covered under provincial health plans. Surgery is the only definitive method of detecting ovarian cancer.

PRESCRIPTION FOR HEALTH

Nutrient	Dosage	Action
Multivitamin with minerals, *no iron* FemmEssentials or MultiEssentials for women	As directed See Appendix A for complete formula recommendations	Ensures adequate nutrient status

Milk Thistle	50-100 mg daily	Supports liver health, which is important for metabolism of hormones
Calcium D-glucarate	150-300 mg daily	Important for healthy metabolism of estrogen; stops abnormal cell growth
Turmeric (95% curcumin)	50-100 mg daily	Prevents abnormal cell growth, detoxifies cancer-causing form of estrogen
Indole-3-carbinol (found in cruciferous vegetables)	150-300 mg daily	Eliminates excess toxic and cancer-causing estrogens. Has been shown to reverse abnormal PAP tests within 3 menstrual cycles
Chaste Tree (Vitex) berry	100-175 mg daily	Balances estrogen-to-progesterone ratio, important for proper cell function. Normalizes ovulation and prolactin
Evening Primrose oil	3000 mg per day	Anti-inflammatory; controls negative prostaglandins involved in pain and inflammation
Green tea extract	100-200 mg daily	Protects against abnormal cell growth, detoxifies excess estrogens
Rosemary extract	25-50 mg daily	Reduces tumor formation; is antioxidant
Lycopene	5-10 mg daily	Antioxidant; reduces risk of cancer
Sulforaphane (found in cruciferous vegetables)	100 mcg-200 mcg daily	Reduces risk of cancer; stops abnormal cell growth

Natural progesterone cream	In Canada, progesterone cream is a prescription drug. Use 6% natural progesterone 1/4 to 1/2 tsp morning and night between days 5-28 (or whenever your normal cycle ends). In the U.S., ProgestaCare by Life Flo is nice as it delivers 20 mg in a pre-measured pump dose.	Limits abnormal cell growth caused by too much estrogen. Aids ovulation

HEALTH TIPS TO ENHANCE HEALING

■ *See* health tips for Endometriosis.

■ Weight loss is essential in those with polycystic ovarian syndrome. *See* Diabetes for tips on normalizing insulin and improving insulin resistance, which aids PCOS.

Overweight and Obesity

Obesity and being overweight constitute the second leading cause of preventable death, after smoking, and are considered to be the most common nutritional disorders in the industrialized world today. More than 60 percent of the U.S. population has a weight problem. The picture is much the same in Canada with data provided by the Canadian Community Health Survey between 1990 and 2001 showing that 48 percent of the Canadian population is packing too much poundage and 15 percent is classified as obese.

Pharmaceutical companies are pumping billions of dollars into new weight-loss drugs to fight the war against fat. Geneticists try to unlock and manipulate the genes that make us fat—one day hoping for a vaccine that will keep us thin. Yet the secret, as you will discover in this section, may be more complicated than reducing calories and exercising more often—our hormones may be the culprits contributing to our fatness.

Causes

Old theories about weight loss were based on the "calories in, calories out" rhetoric. Simply put, if you ate less food and exercised more, weight loss would occur. Those who exercise daily, eat salad and carrot sticks, drink glass after glass of water and still don't lose weight can vouch that weight loss is not that simple. And we all know the person who can eat whatever they wish, has never set foot on a treadmill and doesn't put on a pound. There is a complex interplay of hormonal, biochemical, genetic, physical and lifestyle factors that are causing our battle of the bulge.

You know you have to exercise but you have no "get up and go." Low thyroid function and exhausted adrenals are two other reasons why we gain weight and have no desire to work out. *See* Adrenal Exhaustion and Thyroid for more information.

Basal Metabolic Rate: Your Basal Metabolic Rate (BMR) is the rate at which your body burns calories when you are at rest. Thyroid hormones and how much you exercise are two factors, among many, that have an effect on what your metabolic rate is when you are doing nothing. Metabolism refers to the chemical reactions that take place inside our cells to create energy. All the fuel, which includes carbohydrates, fats, essential fats and proteins, in the food we eat is broken down to produce the energy the body needs to maintain our body temperature, help us breathe, move our muscles and more. A peak operating metabolism can burn up a lot of fuel (food) and create plenty of energy or conversely a slow metabolism will store the fuel as fat. Thermogenesis is the process that burns stored fat.

Liver Function: If you have been dieting for years and were never told a healthy liver is essential for fat loss it isn't any wonder you may not have reached your fat-loss goals. The liver is the most important organ in the body, filtering blood, processing and packaging hormones, removing toxins, metabolizing proteins and carbohydrates into energy, manufacturing cholesterol and breaking down fats, among hundreds of other vital functions.

Excess weight around the middle, whites of the eyes that are dotted with fatty yellow bumps, fatty cysts and skin mottled with "age spots" are all signs of a congested liver, more commonly called a "fatty liver." Clogged bile ducts, inadequate secretion of bile, not enough bile, or an overwhelmed or congested liver from too many prescription drugs, toxins or alcohol can all contribute to a fatty liver. These factors cause our liver to inadequately break down or emulsify fats, and our fat cells to store too much fat, promoting weight gain or resistance to fat loss.

Hormones That Make Us Fat: Any disruption of the liver detoxification pathway contributes to excesses or imbalances in hormones, toxins and our ability to lose weight. The liver is also responsible for conjugating or combining estrogens and other steroid hormones, certain drugs and chemical compounds. Too much estrogen (also called estrogen dominance) is one reason why women have a difficult time losing fat around the abdominal area. A decreased rate of estrogen excretion via liver detoxification contributes to what we commonly call "estrogen belly," which is simply too much fat around the middle, promoted by too much estrogen due to faulty excretion of excess estrogens.

Too much fat on our body also increases our estrogen levels as fat cells are a storage site for estrogen. Contributing to our fatness is the fact that fat cells also manufacture estrogen. This sets up a viscous cycle of too many fat cells manufacturing and storing too much estrogen which creates high levels of estrogen which maintains our increased fat.

Insulin, a hormone secreted by the pancreas, may be the main culprit contributing to our "fatness." The standard excessively high carbohydrate, low protein diet is disrupting our body's ability to regulate blood sugar adequately. When we have too much insulin being pumped out to reduce abnormally high blood sugar, we inevitably gain weight, become fat and our cells become very resistant to insulin and fat loss. Everyone who is overweight has insulin resistance and insulin resistance puts us at higher risk of heart disease, cancers and diabetes.

Another deadly aspect of high insulin is that it increases the secretion of cortisol, our stress hormone. High cortisol causes a corresponding drop in the hormone dehydroepiandrosterone (DHEA). DHEA helps to increase muscle mass, improve immune function, is a precursor to other hormones and has been called our anti-aging hormone. Most importantly for fat loss, we know that more muscle mass causes increased fat burning and a reduction in insulin. As we can see, high insulin promotes a very negative cascade of effects.

Leptin, a hormone produced by body fat, is critical in telling the body when to eat and when we are satisfied. We know that in some people the message of satiety is not heard and the fat cells send out more and more leptin, causing resistance to leptin, increased food cravings and the desire to continue eating. In other people, leptin levels are low due to zinc deficiency.

Unrelenting chronic stress is another factor that promotes weight gain. New research performed at Laval University in Quebec shows that chronic stress causes our fat cells to become resistant to fat loss, especially fat cells around our abdomens. Cortisol activates fat cells—all fat cells—to store fat! But those that are called central fat cells, found mainly deep in the abdominal wall, have four times the cortisol receptors on their cell membranes. Each time you are stressed the cortisol-fat mechanism turns on and your body stores more fat to handle all the stress you are experiencing.

Serotonin, a neurotransmitter in the brain made from the amino acids found in proteins, is also involved in notifying your brain that you are satisfied and can put down your fork. Neurotransmitters are messengers that communicate between cells. Low serotonin causes depression, obesity, lethargy and a preference for refined carbohydrates and overeating because the brain senses it is starving. Those that are hyper-secretors of cortisol exhibit suppressed serotonin levels, which may lead to problems managing weight. We know that in vulnerable persons depression promotes weight gain. When we diet and restrict protein-rich calories, our serotonin levels also plummet. The connection between serotonin, cortisol and weight gain is currently being heavily researched. Simply by lowering cortisol levels through stress management and the use of specific serotonin-enhancing nutritional supplements, including 5-HTP (5-hydroxytryptophan), you can begin to regain control over your weight.

PRESCRIPTION FOR HEALTH

Nutrient	Dosage	Action
Multivitamin with minerals (FemmEssentials or MultiEssentials)	As directed. See Appendix A for complete formula recommendations	For optimal nutrient status. To aid proper thyroid function and support adrenals Contains zinc, known to normalize leptin

		• Contains essential fatty acids including GLA and flaxseed oil to aid metabolism of fat
ThyroSense if you suspect low thyroid is contributing to your weight problem	2 capsules once or twice daily. Ensure your total daily iodine from all sources does not exceed 300 to 400 mcg.	Important for enhancing metabolic rate for proper weight loss. Support for the thyroid gland.
Phase 2 (Phaseolamin)	500 mg-1000 mg a day before meals	Blocks up to 80 percent of starch eaten at a meal.
Cassia nomame	75 mg per day before meals	Reduces fat absorption by up to 30 percent at a meal
Gymnena sylvestra	50 mg per day before meals	Improves the action of insulin and reduces fasting blood sugar levels, to improve overall blood sugar control.
Citrus Aurantium	150-325 mg per day	A natural stimulant, Citrus aurantium supplies synephrine which is a thermogenic known to increase metabolism rate to burn fat more efficiently. Improves energy levels during aerobic exercise, allowing you to work out longer and with more endurance
Garcinia cambogia (Citrimax)	500-2000 mg per day Also available as a tea	Helps to halt the conversion of carbohydrates into fat and increase fat-releasing enzymes. It also inhibits glucose-stimulated insulin secretion.
Green tea extract	200 mg per day	Thermogenic action aids fat loss. Helps control blood sugar levels

Cayenne pepper	100 mg per day	Thermogenic action aids fat loss.
CLA	4000-6000 mg	Burns fat
5-HTP	50-100 mg three times daily	Stops carbohydrate cravings. Improves mood
Protein powder (ProteinEssentials)	2 scoops, 30 grams daily	Revs up fat burning. Contains amino acids including tyrosine which binds with iodine to make thyroid hormones

HEALTH TIPS

- In addition, I recommend you look for my new book *The Body Sense Natural Diet* (Wiley 2004) or visit my website at www.hormonehelp.com
- To rev up your fat-burning furnace, eat protein for breakfast. This will increase your metabolism by 25 percent and that increase lasts for several hours.
- Quantity of food is given most of the credit for our weight woes; the quality of the food we eat plays an equally important role. Saturated fats, trans-fats, fake fats, aspartame and other artificial sweeteners, refined carbohydrates, processed meats and cheese, diet foods and sodas conspire to make us fat and disrupt our hormones. Eliminate all of these toxic foods.
- Have your thyroid checked. *See* Thyroid.
- Use PGX™ fiber in Slim Styles and BodySense Meal Replacements.
- Keep insulin levels normal by eating small, protein-rich meals throughout the day and eliminating the white foods (white sugar, white flour, white rice, white pasta, white potatoes). *See* Diabetes.
- Allergies and sensitivities to food also contribute to increased bloating, poor digestion, weight gain, water retention and an overall puffy appearance. Leaky gut syndrome is caused by years of food allergies, bacterial overgrowth in the gut, *Candida* and stress (high cortisol). The name "leaky gut" refers to when waste, bacteria, and partially digested food are allowed to pass into the bloodstream from a damaged or leaky gut. The foreign substances that should have stayed in our digestive system are now floating in the bloodstream, causing additional stress on the liver and fluid retention, with some individuals packing around 10 to 15 pounds of extra fluids. Our body is approximately two-thirds water,

found in all our cells and tissues (where it is essential for all bodily functions). But when water becomes trapped in tissues and around cells, detoxification and proper cell function, including the movement of fat into and out of cells is inhibited.

■ Exercise 10 minutes with weights every day.

Precocious Puberty

According to medical texts, the average age of the beginning of sexual maturation for females is around age eleven with breast budding, and first menstruation occurs around age thirteen. For some girls, however, sexual maturation comes early, and is considered precocious when the process begins before age eight. Remember from the section on breast cancer that early menstruation is a risk factor for breast cancer as well.

Symptoms

True precocious puberty involves the development of both the exterior and organ changes associated with adulthood, while pseudo-precocious puberty refers to changes in the outward appearance only. Breast development, pubic and underarm hair, changes in body odor and acne might develop. In many girls menstruation also occurs. An early growth spurt typically results in an early stopping of growth, and a shorter final height than anticipated in girls with precocious puberty. Girls who develop precocious puberty need to be continually monitored for low levels of thyroid hormones.

Causes

Sometimes a tumor or other abnormality in the pituitary or hypothalamus can cause the condition, but this only accounts for about 20 percent of the cases of precocious puberty in girls over the age of six. Low thyroid hormone levels may be another factor responsible for precocious puberty. Some doctors also theorize that low birth weight causes a rapid "catch-up phase" that triggers early puberty, while others suggest that North Americans are over-eating and under-exercising, causing additional fat that stores estrogen. A 2002 study linked female obesity with the onset of early puberty. In North America, one in four children between the ages of two and five are obese. Diets lacking in fruits and vegetables also do not provide sufficient fiber, which is necessary for pulling excess estrogen from the body.

Complicating our internal hormone environment are the numerous hormones that are injected into the meats and become part of the dairy products that we feed our children. In addition, estrogen mimickers, technically known as xenoestrogens (pronounced zeno-estrogens) are found in everything from plastic toys to food, cleaning agents to medical supplies. Similar to estrogen in structure, these chemicals bind to estrogen receptor sites throughout the body and cause the same reactions as estrogen would. Young girls who are fascinated with sparkly make-up and perfumes are also exposed to xenoestrogens every time they play dress-up, as most cosmetic products contain estrogen-like compounds. Research is now linking certain chemicals to the development of early puberty in girls.

Diets high in processed foods and refined sugars congest the liver, the large intestine, the colon and the kidneys. With so many toxins to process, these organs cannot possibly neutralize additional estrogen mimickers in our bodies.

PRESCRIPTION FOR HEALTH

Nutrient	Dosage	Action
Multivitamin with minerals; *no iron* FemmEssentials or MultiEssentials for women	As directed See Appendix A for nutrient profile	Ensures adequate nutrient status
Milk Thistle	25 mg daily	Supports liver health, which is important for metabolism of hormones
Calcium D-glucarate	75 mg daily	Important for healthy metabolism of estrogen; supports normal cell growth

Turmeric (95% curcumin)	25 mg daily	Prevents abnormal cell growth, detoxifies cancer-causing form of estrogen
Indole-3-carbinol (found in cruciferous vegetables)	75 mg daily	Stops healthy estrogen from converting into the cancer-causing form. Has been shown to reverse abnormal PAP tests within 3 menstrual cycles
Chaste Tree (Vitex) berry	50 to 100 mg daily	Balances estrogen-to-progesterone ratio important for proper cell function
Evening Primrose oil	500 mg per day	Anti-inflammatory; controls negative prostaglandins involved in pain and inflammation
Green tea extract	50 mg daily	Protects against abnormal cell growth, detoxifies excess estrogens
Rosemary extract	12.5 mg daily	Reduces tumor formation; antioxidant
Lycopene	2.5 mg daily	Antioxidant; reduces risk of cancer
Sulforaphane (found in cruciferous vegetables)	100 mcg daily	Reduces risk of cancer; stops abnormal cell growth
Omega 3 from Flax oil or fish oil	Use flax oil on salads or take Learning Factors™ as directed	Supports healthy cell growth
Acidophilus	found in good yogurts	Builds good bacteria in the digestive tract

HEALING HEALTH TIPS

- See Endometriosis and Breast Cancer for more information on how to eliminate xenoestrogens from the diet and household.
- Avoid microwaving foods in plastic wrap as this leaches xenoestrogens into the food.
- Eat a predominantly vegetarian diet with seven to ten servings of fresh produce daily, and 25 g of fiber to help naturally eliminate estrogen. Girls who are brought up on a complete vegetarian diet get their menstrual cycles later than those who eat a high meat or dairy product diet.
- Consume only organically farmed meat, fish and produce to reduce the chemical burden in your body.
- Include essential fatty acids from fish, flax, nuts and seeds.
- Our children should take a multivitamin with minerals once they are weaned and throughout their lives.
- Do not use bubble bath and personal care products that contain pthalates, parabens and other toxic chemicals.

Premenstrual Syndrome

Premenstrual syndrome (PMS) is the brunt of many terrible jokes, yet this syndrome can be devastating to the sufferer and her family. The symptoms of PMS affect between 50 percent and 70 percent of women, leading to the mistaken belief that it is normal. Symptoms can occur at different times and at different intensities throughout the cycle, but typically appear between seven and fourteen days before menstruation. I am continually amazed at how many women think that PMS and terrible periods are an inevitable part of being female, even though common PMS is not normal.

Symptoms

Symptoms of PMS range from swollen and tender breasts, altered sex drive and uterine cramps to bloating, constipation and diarrhea with a change in appetite and cravings for carbohydrates and other foods. Other symptoms include backaches, water retention, fatigue and insomnia, heart palpitations, dizziness, headaches and migraine, skin problems, herpes and other signs of reduced immunity. Most people associate PMS with moodiness, anxiety, irritability or depression. One of the hallmark symptoms is angry outbursts that are difficult for the sufferer to control, hence its categorization as a psychiatric condition or hysteria.

Causes

PMS is linked to liver and bowel congestion, poor diet and lack of exercise. Hormonal imbalances are also a factor, and may involve estrogen excess; an excess or deficiency in progesterone; thyroid imbalances; high levels of aldosterone, an adrenal hormone that can cause muscle spasms; or prolactin excess. Some research suggests that increased estrogen is associated with decreased serotonin, the "feel good" hormone. Serotonin helps to regulate mood, and a deficiency is linked to depression.

Deficiencies or excess prostaglandins can also lead to PMS symptoms. Prostaglandins are hormone-like substances that regulate a range of physiological responses, including inflammation and muscle contraction, along with some reproductive functions.

Deficiencies in nutrients such as magnesium, vitamins A and E and B-complex, particularly B6, can also be a factor in PMS. Those with PMS often eat more refined sugars, carbohydrates, salt and dairy. Vegetarian women tend to experience less PMS, suggesting a link with meat and dairy consumption (they contain high levels of xenoestrogens). Women who suffer from PMS also tend to have low levels of gamma linolenic acid (GLA) and other essential fats.

PRESCRIPTION FOR HEALTH

Nutrient	Dosage	Action
Multivitamin with minerals, *no iron* FemmEssentials or MultiEssentials for women	As directed. See Appendix A for complete formula recommendations	Ensures adequate nutrient status. B vitamins are essential to treating PMS along with a foundation of good nutrients

Milk Thistle	50-100 mg daily	Supports liver health, which is important for metabolism of hormones
Calcium D-glucarate	150-300 mg daily	Important for healthy metabolism of estrogen; supports normal cell growth
Turmeric (95% curcumin)	50-100 mg daily	Prevents abnormal cell growth; detoxifies cancer-causing forms of estrogen
Indole-3-carbinol (found in cruciferous vegetables)	150-300 mg daily	Normalizes the estrogen-to progesterone-ratios, helping to reduce PMS symptoms. Keeps healthy estrogen from converting into the cancer-causing form. Has been shown to reverse abnormal PAP tests within 3 menstrual cycles
Chaste Tree (Vitex) berry	100-175 mg daily	Balances estrogen-to-progesterone ratio. Reduces and/or eliminates PMS symptoms. Normalizes prolactin levels.
Evening Primrose oil	3000 mg per day	Effective in halting symptoms of PMS. Anti-inflammatory; controls negative prostaglandins involved in pain and inflammation
Green tea extract	100-200 mg daily	Protects against abnormal cell growth; detoxifies excess estrogens
Rosemary extract	25-50 mg daily	Reduces tumor formation; antioxidant; important for healthy thyroid function

Lycopene	5-10 mg daily	Antioxidant, reduces risk of cancer
Sulforaphane (found in cruciferous vegetables)	200-400 mcg daily	Reduces risk of cancer; stops abnormal cell growth; helps balance hormones
Natural progesterone cream	In Canada, progesterone cream is a prescription drug. Use 6% natural progesterone 1/4 to1/2 tsp morning and night between days 5-28 (or whenever your normal cycle ends). In the U.S., ProgestaCare by Life Flo is nice as it delivers 20 mg in a pre-measured pump dose.	Improves the ratio of progesterone to estrogen. Limits the endometrial tissue build-up caused by estrogen. Ensure proper monitoring (blood and saliva tests) is done so you do not develop progesterone excess
Omega-6 fatty acids	Evening Primrose oil 4000 mg per day or Borage oil 2000 mg per day	GLA found in evening primrose and borage oil helps control inflammatory prostaglandins, and reduces breast tenderness
5-HTP 5-hydroxy-tryptophan	50-100 mg three times per day.	Enhances serotonin ("feel good" hormone), improves mood, calms anxiety and nervousness, helps mild depression; improves sleep

HEALTH TIPS TO ENHANCE HEALING

- *See* Endometriosis, Fibrocystic Breasts and Menopause health tips.
- Peri-menopause and menopause can be a time when women experience the most severe PMS symptoms.
- Have your thyroid checked. Low thyroid hormone levels create severe PMS symptoms.
- Eliminate all xenoestrogens from the diet and home.
- Cut back on caffeine from all sources (chocolate, soda pop, coffee and black tea). Drink herbal tea.

- A high-fiber diet with plenty of organic fruits and vegetables helps to eliminate excess estrogen.
- Eat only organic meats, and eliminate dairy from the diet. Both contain high amounts of xenoestrogens.
- Meditation, exercise and acupuncture are techniques help reduce the symptoms of PMS. Love yourself. Get plenty of rest. You do not have to be the "super" mom, wife and employee.

Thyroid (Hypothyroidism)

Hypothyroidism or low thyroid hormone is a common condition in North America, particularly Canada and the upper U.S. states where levels of sunlight are low for much of the year, and soil mineral depletion is common. Low thyroid function affects approximately 20-25 percent of the female population and about 10 percent of males. An additional 30 percent of persons over the age of 35 may also have sub-clinical or mild hypothyroidism whereby their thyroid stimulating hormone (TSH) is within normal range, but they have many of the symptoms of low thyroid. The thyroid secretes two hormones—T3 and T4—that are crucial for controlling our metabolism. Because thyroid hormones affect every cell in the body, a deficiency will result in many symptoms.

The thyroid is a small gland that lies below the Adam's apple in the neck, wrapped around both sides of the trachea. It secretes thyroid hormones that control many metabolic functions in the body. Thyroid hormones stimulate the production of proteins and increase the use of oxygen by cells in the body. Iodine is required by the thyroid to produce thyroid hormones. A careful recycling process occurs in the thyroid to ensure adequate thyroid hormones are available to control the body's metabolic rate. The following hormones and substances directly affect the thyroid or are released by it:

- Thyrotropin releasing hormone (TRH) is secreted by the hypothalamus, a brain centre that coordinates the actions of the nervous and endocrine systems. TRH triggers the pituitary to secrete TSH.
- Thyroid stimulating hormone (TSH) is secreted by the pituitary in response to TRH. TSH stimulates the production of thyroid hormones and the growth

of thyroid cells (excess TSH causes thyroid enlargement, or goiter.)

- Calcitonin is a thyroid hormone involved in the homeostasis of blood calcium levels. It lowers the amount of calcium and phosphate in the blood as needed by inhibiting bone breakdown and accelerating the assimilation of calcium. Thus, the thyroid is involved in bone health and diseases such as osteoporosis.
- Thyroxin (T4) is the most abundant thyroid hormone and is manufactured in the thyroid gland. It is synthesized from tyrosine and includes four molecules of iodine per molecule of thyroxin hormone.
- Triiodothyronine (T3) is the most active thyroid hormone, with four to ten times the activity of T4. It includes three molecules of iodine per molecule of hormone. Twenty percent of T3 is produced and secreted by the thyroid gland and the other 80 percent is converted from T4 in the liver and other organs. Many factors contribute to the conversion of T4 to the more active T3, including liver health, low stress levels, the types of foods you consume and more.

At any given time, most T3 and T4 molecules in the body are bound tightly to blood proteins. Only a small amount of each circulates as "free" hormone that is physiologically active. For example, unbound T4 accounts for approximately 0.05 percent of total T4. Unbound hormone levels are seldom measured by medical doctors, yet these levels are most accurate for determining thyroid function.

A delicate balance must be maintained to keep a steady metabolic rate in the body. The hypothalamus and pituitary glands work in concert with the proteins of the body, T4, the liver and other organs to maintain that balance.

When the thyroid produces too much thyroid hormone, hyperthyroidism develops. Autoimmune reactions against the thyroid can cause hyperthyroidism; Graves' disease is one such condition. The immune system malfunctions, causing an increase in thyroid hormone. Goiter, a greatly enlarged thyroid gland, is seen in those with Graves' disease and is due to the excessive secretion of thyroid hormone. Thyroiditis, an inflammation of the thyroid gland, can initially cause hyperthyroidism, but eventually the damage to the thyroid caused by the inflammation causes hypothyroidism or low thyroid function.

Low Thyroid Function, Peri-menopause, Menopause and Weight Gain: Estrogen decides body fat distribution, and, in women, fat is stored on our hips, bottom, abdomen and thighs. Fat cells manufacture and store estrogen. Some researchers believe women get an increase in body fat around menopause to ensure adequate estrogen from fat cells. Others believe that it is low thyroid and exhausted adrenals that promote mid-section fat gain. Considering that excess fat reduces our life expectancy, I tend to believe the latter because the body is generally programmed to ensure our survival.

I mentioned earlier that there could be as high as 30 percent of people over the age of 35 walking around with sub-clinical low thyroid function. We know that low thyroid function promotes many hormonal problems that could be remedied with thyroid-supporting nutrients or medication (thyroid hormones).

During the peri-menopausal years (the 10 to 15 years before menopause) and menopause (menopause means one year with no periods), it is common for women to suffer a multitude of hormonal complaints. Hot flashes, night sweats and sleep disturbances are common complaints during this time in a woman's life. Most would think these symptoms are associated with a decline in estrogen, but they are also hallmark symptoms of low thyroid, especially night sweats and insomnia. Most menopausal women are given hormone replacement therapy with estrogen for these symptoms. Peri-menopausal women may be put on the birth control pill. The problem with these treatments is that estrogen further shuts down the thyroid: high estrogen levels interfere with the thyroid hormones, particularly the utilization of T3, the most biologically active thyroid hormone. I have to reiterate that too much estrogen either from hormone replacement therapy or your own estrogen causes a host of problems and also impairs thyroid function.

Many women have experienced a ten-to 15-pound weight gain and increased blood pressure when they started taking synthetic estrogen at menopause. This happens because estrogen is an antagonist to thyroid hormone and the metabolic rate slows down. As this happens, many women develop difficulties with fat metabolism, because one of the functions of the thyroid hormones is to stimulate fat cells to burn fat. Weight control problems result.

In addition, serum cholesterol or triglyceride levels may increase. Thyroid activity can also be inhibited by high levels of androgens (male sex hormones) circulating in the blood. Depression and fatigue are the most common thyroid symptoms in menopausal women.

Many people suffer with mild or sub-clinical low thyroid function—their thyroid stimulating hormone (TSH, the hormone that stimulates your thyroid to make thyroid hormones) is greater than 2.0 IU/ml but less than the 5.5 IU/ml level indicative of hypothyroidism. As such they contend with the many symptoms of low thyroid function but are not being treated with medication. If you are trying to lose weight and have followed a healthy eating plan and exercised and still cannot lose a pound, you may have sub-clinical low thyroid function.

Many people's TSH falls within the conventional parameters for normal (0.3 to 6.0), but most people with levels greater than 2.0 have symptoms of low thyroid function. Enlightened doctors refer to such people as having sub-clinical, or functional, low thyroid function.

If a diagnosis of low thyroid is based solely on a TSH reading, without taking other symptoms into account, it may take ten years before thyroid hormone levels drop low enough to trigger a mainstream diagnosis of low thyroid function. In the meantime, the person with low thyroid function symptoms will go through much unnecessary suffering.

Low Thyroid Function and Hormonal Problems: It is common for the thyroid to be functionally, or even clinically, out of balance in women who experience hormone-related problems such as premenstrual syndrome (PMS), infertility, ovarian cysts, fibroids, endometriosis, fibrocystic breasts, dysmenorrhea (menstrual pain), metrorrhagia (heavy bleeding) or menopausal symptoms. Back in the days before fertility drugs, when a woman could not get pregnant or had recurring miscarriages, doctors prescribed thyroid hormone with some success. Women who suffer post-partum depression could also benefit from thyroid hormone as childbearing can often exhaust the adrenals and promote low thyroid.

Symptoms

The symptoms of hypothyroidism are varied. Hypothyroidism causes the body's metabolic rate to slow dramatically, and early symptoms are often misdiagnosed as depression. Slowed heart rate, hoarse voice, slowed speech, swollen and puffy face, drooping eyelids, intolerance to cold, constipation and weight gain are hallmark symptoms. The hair often becomes sparse, coarse and dry and there is a loss of eyebrow hair. The skin will become dry, scaly, thick and bumpy and may have raised thickened areas on the shins. Carpal tunnel syndrome, muscle weakness, confusion, depression, dementia, heart disease with high cholesterol and triglyceride levels, hormone disruptions, shortness of breath and extreme fatigue may also be present. Women with hypothyroidism may also experience heavy menstrual bleeding, infertility and, when they do become pregnant, they are at increased risk of miscarriages, premature deliveries and stillbirths.

Have your thyroid function checked by your doctor, but don't be surprised if the results come back normal even though you have a large number of the symptoms above. Many people have sub-clinical low thyroid and yet are diagnosed with normal thyroid based on the current tests. The Barnes basal temperature test can better help determine thyroid function. This simple temperature test can determine if you have low thyroid. Men and non-menstruating women can take the test on any day, but women who are menstruating should take the test on the second, third or fourth day of their period. (*See* Thyroid Basal Temperature Home Test in Appendix C)

Those women with low thyroid are at serious health risk for many other conditions. As well, nutritional therapies do not work as well in those with an under-active thyroid.

Causes
Hashimoto's thyroiditis is the most common cause of hypothyroidism. The autoimmune process attacks the thyroid and eventually the thyroid cannot produce enough thyroid hormone. The treatment of hyperthyroidism, using radioactive iodine and surgery, is the second most common cause of hypothyroidism.

Decades ago, iodine was added to salt to make iodized salt to treat goiter and subsequent thyroid problems, but many people are no longer eating salt and, as a result, we are seeing an increase in hypothyroidism. As well, stress, anemia, estrogen replacement, birth control pills and other medications that block iodine uptake are associated with an increase in hypothyroidism.

Those living in the northern hemisphere are not getting enough sunshine to produce vitamin D, a cofactor in thyroid hormone production; as a result they are more prone to hypothyroidism. Trace minerals are also required to make thyroid hormone, and deficiencies promote hypothyroidism.

PRESCRIPTION FOR HEALTH

You should not stop your thyroid medication—it is essential for providing adequate thyroid hormone. If you are on medication but still have the symptoms of low thyroid function, add the following nutrients for better conversion of T4 to the more active T3. Recommendations below are designed to support thyroid function.

Nutrient	Dosage	Action
Multivitamin with minerals (FemmEssentials or MultiEssentials)	As directed. See Appendix A for complete formula recommendations	For optimal nutrient status. Required for thyroid, metabolism and for proper immune function
Potassium Iodide	100 mg one to two times daily. Ensure your total daily iodine from all sources does not exceed 300-400 mcg.	Iodine's only role in the body is to make thyroid hormones. Too little causes impaired thyroid function; too much iodine interferes with the thyroid's ability to make thyroid hormones. Important for fertility, fibrocystic breasts, breast cancer prevention, and to destroy H. pylori in the gut and more
Tyrosine (amino acid)	500 mg one to two times daily	A key component in the function of the thyroid gland
Ashwagandha	150 mg one to two times daily	Increases T4 thyroid hormone. Acts directly on the thyroid gland.
Commiphora mukul extract (Gugguls)	100 mg one to two times daily	Enhances the conversion of T4 to the more active T3. Works synergistically with Ashwagandha directly on the thyroid gland

Pantothenic acid	100 mg one to two times daily	Supports adrenal glands; increases energy; helps you handle stress better. Added benefit: works to combat cellulite.
Copper	500 mcg one to two times daily	Support for the thyroid gland
Manganese	500 mcg one to two times daily	Support for the thyroid gland
Protein powder (ProteinEssentials containing tyrosine)	2 scoops, 30 g daily	Contains amino acids, including tyrosine which binds with iodine to make thyroid hormones

HEALTH TIPS TO ENHANCE HEALING

- Reduce your consumption of foods (called goitrogens) that impede the absorption of iodine, if you have hypothyroidism. These foods include soy, turnips, cabbage, mustard greens, peanuts, pine nuts and millet. You would have to eat these foods every day to impede thyroid hormone, but just as a precaution be aware of their effects.

- Dessicated Thyroid should be taken under the guidance of your physician.

- Avoid fluoride toothpaste and fluoridated water as they compete with iodine for absorption.

- Ensure you get adequate sunshine. The thyroid gland requires vitamin D to function properly. Those living in the northern hemisphere have higher rates of low thyroid. Take ThyroSense to support thyroid health. *See* www. thyrosense.com

- Detoxification and elimination of waste is very important. Eat liver-friendly foods such as kale, carrots, beets, artichokes, lemons, onions, garlic, leeks.

- Stress reduction is essential. *See* Adrenal Exhaustion. The adrenals and the thyroid are linked. If the adrenals are exhausted, low thyroid hormones will result. If you have low thyroid function, it promotes stress on the adrenals.

- If you are having fertility problems, ensure your doctor does sensitive thyroid tests to rule out sub-clinical low thyroid function. A fertility clinic in Toronto found that 25 percent of its patients had low thyroid function that was not detected on the standard TSH test. *See* Thyroid Tests in Appendix C.

- Severe hypothyroidism, confirmed by a thyroid stimulating hormone (TSH) test, requires the use of thyroid medication. Most medical doctors prefer the synthetic thyroid hormone T4, but some physicians and patients prefer desiccated natural thyroid obtained from the glands of animals (mainly pigs). Desiccated thyroid also contains the more active T3. When initially prescribed it may be difficult for some people to get the correct dose of desiccated thyroid medicine unless your doctor is willing to monitor your TSH, T3 and T4 adequately. This is a problem in Canada where medical doctors are not as familiar with natural hormones and where the medical system will only pay for certain diagnostic tests and only so many per year. Desiccated thyroid is available through compounding pharmacies in Canada.

Urinary Tract Infections and Interstitial Cystitis

Urinary Tract Infections

Infections of the bladder, urethra and kidneys are known as urinary tract infections (UTIs). Because the urethra is so close to the anus in females, women experience UTIs twice as often as men. UTIs must be treated promptly as they can cause permanent damage to the urinary tract. An infection in the bladder is called cystitis, while pyelonephritis is a more serious infection located in the kidneys. Urine tests are often used to diagnose UTI, but women are prone to symptoms of UTI without the presence of bacteria in the urine. Interstitial cystitis is one such condition, affecting more than one million North Americans. The continual inflammation from the infection results in a shrunken bladder that causes frequent urination, and pain that can interfere with sexual activity and may lead to depression.

Symptoms

UTIs involve more frequent urination, with associated pain and burning. Urine may be darker or contain blood, and have an odor. Fever or flu-like symptoms are common, and pain in the lower back often accompanies a kidney infection.

Causes

Most UTIs are caused by bacteria that have transferred from the anus or vagina to the urethra. Some known risks are antibiotic use, stress, sexual contact, oral contraceptives, diaphragms, diabetes, a weakened immune system or hormonal imbalances during menopause. *Candida* overgrowth is another factor, as are parasites.

Interstitial Cystitis

Interstitial cystitis is a chronic inflammation of the urinary bladder lining and the bladder muscle. While there is no bladder autoantigen that has been identified, it is similar enough to lupus and coincides often enough with it and other autoimmune disorders that it is discussed in the field of autoimmunity. Predominantly a female affliction, only ten percent of interstitial cystitis cases occur in men.

It is much more rare, but not out of the question, that children can be afflicted with interstitial cystitis. Because it is primarily thought of as an adult disease, there is little research done on its effects on children. In some cases, the disease can begin before children are able to talk, making diagnosis that much more difficult and unlikely.

Symptoms

The early symptom of interstitial cystitis is frequent urination, day or night. In severe cases it can be necessary 60 times in a day. Eventually the need to urinate becomes urgent; there may be blood in the urine and pain or spasms of the abdomen, urethra or vagina. Inflamation reduces the capacity of the bladder and the bladder wall sports scars and hemorrhaged punctures (or "angry scratches"). Sexual activity for both men and women may be curtailed because it is too painful. The lifetime implications on the sex life and the chronic pain can lead to depression ranging from moderate to severe, and has led to suicide. Other symptoms may be present such as migraines, joint or muscle pain, gastrointestinal problems or allergies.

Causes

The cause for interstitial cystitis is unknown. It can appear as a symptom of lupus or endometriosis and be aggravated by food allergies, diet or lifestyle choices.

PRESCRIPTION FOR HEALTH
RECOMMENDED FOR THOSE WITH UTIs

Nutrient	Dosage	Action
Cranberry CranMax whole cranberry containing lignans 34:1 extract	250 mg two to four times daily	Prevents *E. coli* bacteria from adhering to urinary tract; protects stomach lining from *H. pylori*. The lignans in CranMax protects the CP450 system that prevents breast cancer. This system is shut off during antibiotic therapy
Vitamin C, mineral ascorbates including calcium, magnesium, potassium ascorbate	1000 mg twice daily	Antibacterial; supports immune function
BB536 Bifidobacterium longum	1-2 capsules, 5-10 billion active organisms	Improves intestinal flora to fight bacteria, essential for those taking antibiotics
Goldenseal standardized for Berberine content	500 mg per day	Antibacterial; inhibits bacteria from adhering to the bladder wall
Uva ursi tea	1 cup per day	Uva ursi acts as a diuretic, alleviates pain and fights bacteria (*do not use if pregnant)
Multivitamins with minerals (FemmEssentials or MultiEssentials)	As directed. See Appendix A for complete formula recommendations	To provide optimal nutrient support

RECOMMENDED FOR THOSE WITH INTERSTITIAL CYSTITIS

Prerelief® (calcium glycerophosphate)	2 tablets whenever you eat or drink acidic foods or drinks	Research has shown 70% of those with interstitial cystitis report relief from pain; 61% report a decrease in the urgency to urinate.
Gota kola (Centella asiatica)	200 mg twice a day; use standardized extract	Strengthens bladder wall, reduces the formation of scar tissue
Horsetail and Marshmallow tea	1-2 cups per day	Horsetail strengthens bladder wall; marshmallow calms an irritated bladder

HEALTH TIPS TO ENHANCE HEALING

- Drink plenty of water throughout the day. It is the cheapest substance to reduce pain and burning due to UTIs.
- Enhance your immune system by taking your multivitamin with minerals every day.
- Eat plain, probiotic-rich yogurt daily.
- Urinate when your body tells you to. Don't wait—this increases the likelihood of infection.
- Wear cotton underwear.
- Use NatraCare unbleached panty liners, pads and tampons instead of the bleached type commonly sold.
- Position yourself on top during intercourse to reduce the amount of bacteria being pushed into the urethra.
- Urinate immediately after intercourse.
- Do not use douches.
- Take CranMax and BB536 every day for prevention sold as UriSense.
- A 3-14 day course of antibiotics may be prescribed for the treatment of UTIs, yet some researchers believe that natural treatments should be tried first and only if fever and pain persist for several days should antibiotic therapy be prescribed.

Uterine Fibroids

Uterine fibroids (myomas) are non-cancerous growths that occur on the walls of the uterus. Composed of connective tissue and muscle, these round, firm growths can be microscopic or grow to the size of a grapefruit. After appearing in groups, fibroids typically grow slowly. Fast-growing fibroids may be malignant. At least 20 percent of women over age 35 will experience fibroids at some time. Because fibroids are affected by estrogen levels, some growths tend to shrink at menopause. On the other hand, some increase in size at menopause and become malignant. If fibroids become problematic, doctors often prescribe drugs that trigger menopausal symptoms to encourage growths to shrink to a size that can be removed surgically in a procedure called a myomectomy. Without certain lifestyle changes, however, fibroids will return after surgery. In extreme cases, doctors may recommend hysterectomy. (*See* Hysterectomy, Myomectomy and Uterine Ablation in Appendix C)

Symptoms

Some women are surprised to learn during a pelvic examination that they have fibroids as they have experienced no symptoms, even if they have a rather large growth. Others suffer with menstrual problems including heavy, irregular or painful periods and mid-cycle bleeding. Vaginal discharge, pain or bleeding with intercourse, frequent urination, problems with bowel movements and compromised digestion are also involved. Heavy bleeding can cause anemia and fatigue. During pregnancy, fibroids can cause miscarriage, premature delivery or severe loss of blood after the birth.

Causes

Fibroids are caused by excess estrogen. Causes of estrogen dominance include exposure to xenoestrogens, bowel toxicity and liver congestion. Undiagnosed clinical or functional hypothyroidism is frequently a factor.

Nutrient	Dosage	Action
Multivitamin with minerals, *no iron* FemmEssentials or MultiEssentials for women	As directed See Appendix A for nutrient profile	Ensures adequate nutrient status
Milk Thistle	100 mg daily	Supports liver health, which is important for metabolism of hormones
Calcium D-glucarate	300 mg daily	Important for healthy metabolism of estrogen; supports normal cell growth
Turmeric (95% curcumin)	100 mg daily	Prevents abnormal cell growth; detoxifies cancer-causing form of estrogen
Indole-3-carbinol (found in cruciferous vegetables)	300 mg daily	Stops healthy estrogen from converting into the cancer-causing form. Has been shown to reverse abnormal PAP tests within 3 menstrual cycles
Floradix Iron Tonic	1-4 capfuls daily	Does not constipate; enhances iron
Chaste Tree (Vitex) berry	100 to 175 mg daily	Balances estrogen-to-progesterone ratio; important for proper cell function
Evening Primrose oil	3000 mg per day	Anti-inflammatory; controls negative prostaglandins involved in pain and inflammation

Green tea extract	200 mg daily	Protects against abnormal cell growth; detoxifies excess estrogens
Rosemary extract	50 mg daily	Reduces tumor formation; antioxidant
Lycopene	10 mg daily	Antioxidant; reduces risk of cancer
Sulforaphane (found in cruciferous vegetables)	400 mcg daily	Reduces risk of cancer; stops abnormal cell growth
Natural progesterone cream	In Canada, progesterone cream is a prescription drug. Use 6% natural progesterone 1/4 to 1/2 tsp morning and night between days 5-28 (or whenever your normal cycle ends). In the U.S., ProgestaCare by Life Flo is nice as it delivers 20 mg in a pre-measured pump dose.	Limits the endometrial tissue build-up caused by estrogen
Cramp Bark tincture	1/2 teaspoon every 2-4 hours for acute pain	Relaxes the uterus and reduces cramps
Shepard's Purse	50 drops three times daily	Works together with Evening Primrose oil to reduce bleeding

HEALTH TIPS TO ENHANCE HEALING

- *See* Health Tips for Endometriosis, another estrogen-dominant condition.
- Detoxification and elimination of waste is very important. Eat liver-friendly foods such as kale, carrots, beets, artichokes, lemons, onions, garlic, leeks and members of the cabbage family (broccoli, Brussels sprouts, cauliflower).
- Follow a vegetarian diet and increase your soy and fiber intake. Fiber carries estrogen out of the body. Avoid meat products (except fish). Your diet should concentrate on whole grains, fresh fruits and vegetables. Choose organic foods

whenever possible to reduce the burden of xenoestrogens from pesticides.

- Avoid alcohol, dairy products, caffeine (including medications), sugar, chocolate, coffee, tea and soft drinks. Alcohol interferes with liver function and caffeine exacerbates the growths.

- Lose extra pounds—being overweight can increase effects of estrogen on the uterus. Exercise regularly to burn calories, improve circulation and help the detoxification and elimination process.

- Take EstroSense containing Indole-3-carbinol, d-glucarate, sulforaphone, green tea, curcumin, milk thistle, rosemary and lycopene. See www.estrosense.com for more information.

Vaginal Yeast Infections (Candida)

Seventy percent of women will experience at least one vaginal yeast infection during their lives, and 40 percent will have more than one infection. Studies show that 45 percent of vaginal yeast infections are caused by *Candida albicans* or another species of *Candida* fungus. These fungi, or yeast, normally exist in the intestines and vagina in small numbers, but changes in the internal environment can cause them to proliferate, wreaking havoc on various body systems. The fungi produce hormone-like substances that resemble human hormones, and some types have their own hormone receptors. The immune system often produces antibodies against the *Candida*, causing an allergic response to an organism that normally exists in our bodies.

Symptoms
Vaginal itching and irritation and cheesy white discharge with a distinct odor are common symptoms. Urination may be painful. The skin of the vulva may be raw and red. Often, symptoms worsen the week before menstruation.

Causes
Our bodies contain organisms that live in a delicate balance with one another, and *Candida* is normally held in check by "beneficial" bacteria in our bodies. When the beneficial bacteria become outnumbered, however, the stage is set for

Candida overgrowth. Internal environmental changes can be caused by the use of antibiotics, birth control pills, hormone replacement therapy and other steroid medications, drinking chlorinated water, stress, diabetes and poor nutrition with a diet high in sugar. Other contributing factors include multiple pregnancies, smoking and a weakened immune system.

PRESCRIPTION FOR HEALTH*

Nutrient	Dosage	Action
Multivitamins with minerals (FemmEssentials in Canada or MultiEssentials in the U.S.)	As directed; see Appendix A 1000 mg vitamin C 500 mg quercetin three times daily	Anti-inflammatory; anti-bacterial; improves digestion; reduces stress; aids detoxification; supports immunity
Vitamin K	60-80 mcg per day	Restores imbalance caused by antibiotics
Omega-3 Fatty Acids	1000-3000 mg daily Pharmaceutical Grade Fish oil	Protects the integrity of cells; anti-inflammatory
Caprylic acid (enteric coated)	1-2 grams daily with meals	Acts as an anti-fungal
Oil of Oregano	3 drops 3 times a day in juice or water	Powerful anti-fungal
Tea Tree Oil (must be diluted before application, mix with topical anti-fungals)	local application 40% solution for a maximum of five days	Effective for *Candida* vaginitis. Do not apply to broken skin; if irritation occurs, discontinue
High Lignan Flax seed	1-2 tsp daily	Prevents constipation
Berberine (containing herbs including Goldenseal and Oregon Grape)	Use as directed; make sure berberine content is listed on label	Acts as an anti-fungal but if immunity has been built up to it, substitute clove or maitake

Probiotic supplement (look for BB536 strain) providing billions live organisms	As directed on label	Replenishes and boosts intestinal flora
Garlic Factors	1000 mg per day	Natural anti-fungal
Echinacea (Echinamide)	Use as directed on label for 2 weeks	Research shows a 40% drop in the recurrence of *Candida* vaginal infections

* Pregnant women should consult their naturopathic doctor for treatment of Candida overgrowth.

HEALTH TIPS TO ENHANCE HEALING

- The best protection from *Candida* is to boost the immune system. Eat plenty of fruits and vegetables, 7 to 10 half-cup servings daily. Legumes, fish, whole grains, nuts, seeds and their oils will provide your body with balanced nutrition. Avoid eating simple carbohydrates such as white bread, cake, cookies and chips, and too many citrus fruits that create an alkaline environment in the body and allow *Candida* to flourish.
- If *Candida* is a reoccurring problem, switch to a diet that excludes all yeast and sugar (that means fruit, too). Any food that has been aged or fermented should also be eliminated, so no cheese, soy sauce, pickles, raw mushrooms, vinegar or alcohol to name a few. Avoid gluten and eat millet, quinoa and brown rice instead.
- Eat plenty of plain probiotic-rich (look for the words acidophilus or bifidus or bifidobacterium) yogurt to increase the good bacteria population in your intestines. Half a cup to one cup every day will ward off yeast infections and restore balance to the body. If you are taking antibiotics, always supplement with probiotics.
- Choose organic dairy products to avoid hormones and xenoestrogens.
- Drink at least 8 to 10 glasses of pure, filtered water daily. For every juice, caffeine or alcoholic beverage you consume, have another glass of water.
- Do not overeat; it suppresses the immune system.
- Stop smoking.
- Take one or two digestive enzymes before every meal. Do not drink fluids while eating or you will dilute your enzymes.
- If you suspect you have low stomach acid because you have gas, bloating and

digestive distress, take 1 capsule (600 mg) of hydrochloric acid before a large meal. If symptoms worsen, stop—you do not have low stomach acid. If you feel the same or better, increase your dosage by one at your next meal. Keep increasing the dosage up to a maximum of seven capsules or until you feel warmth in your stomach. If you feel the warmth, cut back to a dosage tolerated prior to the feeling. Use fewer capsules for smaller meals.

- Start a diet diary and write down everything you eat and see if there is any correlation to your allergy symptoms. Ask for a referral to an allergy specialist and get tested for possible triggers. Some allergies may only be detected with the help of an ELISA test. Once you know what you are allergic to, avoid those allergens. Have environmental allergens tested as well.

Other Recommendations

- Wear loose white cotton underwear instead of synthetic, and leave the pantyhose in the drawer. Change undergarments daily, and wash them at high temperatures.
- After going to the toilet, wipe front to back to avoid spreading the fungus back to the vagina.
- Take baths instead of showers to ensure that the genital area is washed thoroughly. Make sure that you dry off very well.
- Avoid taking oral contraceptives or steroid medications; they can alter your body's environment to encourage yeast growth.
- Although there is still the need for more research in this area, sexual transmission is being investigated for its role yeast infections. To be safe, use a condom during sex so you don't infect your partner (who then infects you again).
- Reduce your exposure to chemicals, perfumes, dyes, fragrances and scents. When fighting an infection, don't use bubble bath, douches, perfumed toilet paper, deodorized tampons, etc. Soap should be natural as well.
- Mercury toxicity can make the body vulnerable to yeast overgrowth. Have a hair, urine and blood analysis done to determine if that is a factor. If so, avoid exposure to mercury and have dental amalgams removed.
- If you are having four or more vaginal yeast infections in a year, consult your physician or naturopath.
- Not all infections in the vagina are yeast problems, so have sexually transmitted diseases ruled out.

Varicose Veins

Varicose veins are lumpy, bulging, blue veins on the legs. Women get them four times as often as men, and roughly half of the people above the age of 50 have some type of varicose vein (hemorrhoids are a type of varicosity in the veins of the anus). Veins have little valves on the inner walls of the vessel to prevent blood from flowing backwards. Valves can become dysfunctional due to damage to the vein walls. When this occurs, it prevents proper one-way circulation and blood pools in the veins. The extra fluid causes the veins to stretch and bulge.

Although they are visually unappealing, generally, varicose veins are not harmful if they are small and appear close to the surface of the skin. However, if varicose veins are located deeper within the leg, ulcerations, deep-vein blood clots, or bleeding under the skin can occur. In serious cases, there can be complications such as inflammation of the veins (phlebitis), clots that can relocate in the lungs (pulmonary embolism) and leg ulcerations requiring immediate medical attention.

Symptoms
When the veins get sluggish the legs can feel tight, heavy or restless, and there can be aches or leg cramps, pain and swelling. The veins may itch and sores may develop.

Causes
Veins are fragile and pressure caused by being overweight, smoking, pregnancy and occupational environment (either too much standing, sitting or heavy lifting) cause the veins to dilate, leading to damage of the valves. In fact, ten times the normal pressure is forced on the veins if you are standing for many hours. Other factors include: heart or liver disease, constipation, tumors in the abdomen, vitamin C deficiency, birth control pills, hormone replacement therapy and genetic pre-disposition.

PRESCRIPTION FOR HEALTH
Sclerotherapy and surgery by a specialist to remove large and bulging veins can have excellent results. The following recommendations are effective at eliminating spider veins at the surface but larger veins will most often not be eliminated, only reduced in size with symptoms alleviated.

Nutrient	Dosage	Action
Pharmaceutical grade fish oil	3000 mg per day	Relieves constipation and soothes mucous membranes of the entire intestinal tract. Softens stool
Horse Chestnut Seed Extract	100 to 150 mg daily containing escin or Venastat	Increases antioxidant activity, inhibits enzymes that destroy venous walls, and improves venous tone
Ground flax seed (high lignans)	1 to 2 tablespoons daily	Soothes intestinal lining and promotes elimination
Multivitamin with minerals (FemmEssentials for MultiEssentials for women)	As directed. See Appendix A for complete formula recommendations	Supports immune function; potent antioxidant; supports vein integrity; detoxifies liver; prevents deficiency; repairs blood vessel walls; prevents blood clotting and bruising; improves circulation
Bromelain	500-1000 mg after every meal	Anti-inflammatory, shown to prevent hard, lumpy skin around bulging varicose veins
Gotu Kola (Centella asiatica)	30-60 mg of triterpenic acid content twice daily	Enhances connective tissue integrity and increases blood flow
Flavonoids or cyanidins from bilberry or grape seed extract or pycnogenol	150-500 mg per day	Improves the integrity of capillaries, veins and protects collagen from damage in varicose veins. Potent antioxidant effect, antihistamine

HEALTH TIPS TO ENHANCE HEALING

- *See* Constipation
- Reduce weight; even 10 extra pounds puts added pressure on your venous system.
- Eat foods high in fiber.
- Drink at least 8 to 10 glasses of pure, filtered water every day. Water maintains a healthy level of blood volume and prevents constipation.
- Apply Witch Hazel ointment topically twice a day to reduce swelling and tone veins.
- Avoid standing or sitting for long periods. Regular exercise is mandatory for circulation disorders and maintaining weight.
- Stop smoking. Nicotine constricts blood vessels.

Other Recommendations

- When traveling for long periods of time, make sure that you stand up and move around every once in awhile to keep circulation going and prevent blood clots from forming in the veins. Wear loose fitting clothing and drink plenty of water.
- Supportive elastic stockings, specifically for varicose veins, in combination with the above recommendations can dramatically reduce the appearance of unsightly veins.
- Hydrotherapy can alleviate pain and improve circulation. Fill a bathtub full of cold water, get in and walk on the spot for 20 minutes (Use an anti-slip tub mat.) An alternative is to spray cold water on the legs, front and back, for ten seconds every morning in the shower.
- When sitting or lying down, raise the legs above the heart for 20 minutes every day.
- Shift your weight and stand on your toes periodically if you must stand for long periods of time. If you sit at a desk, wiggle your toes and flex your leg muscles to keep blood flowing. Do not cross your legs and avoid putting pressure on your legs.
- Do not scratch veins if they are itchy, or you may cause further damage.

APPENDIX A:

Supplements for Women's Health

EVERY WOMAN NEEDS A MULTIVITAMIN with minerals, along with essential fatty acids from fish, flax seed, evening primrose or borage oil. In the Introduction to this book, I discuss why it is essential that you have a foundation nutrient formula to support all the enzymatic reactions in your body. Look for a multivitamin with minerals that contains the nutrients listed in the nutrition chart in this appendix. This is your foundation formula upon which you add the nutrients as needed for any disease condition you may have. If you take only one supplement, make sure it is a multivitamin with minerals.

Seven Easy Ways to Get the Most from Your Nutritional Supplements

1. Always take your essential nutrients with food. Digestive enzymes and stomach acid are released when we eat food, facilitating the breakdown and assimilation of nutrients.

2. Buy supplements that are either in capsules, soft gels or powder. Poor digestion is commonplace so ensure your multi-nutrient is in the right form so it can be assimilated properly for better absorption. Tablets have been known to go through the digestive system without being broken down.

3. Look for nutrient formulations with the most absorbable form of vitamins and minerals. Good quality supplements always list the form of the vitamin or mineral, for example, calcium as calcium citrate or vitamin B6 as pyridoxal-5-phosphate. Poor quality supplements do not list the form of the ingredient.

4. Choose a formulation that contains betaine HCl and glutamic acid HCl. If you have ever taken vitamins or minerals and felt nauseous afterward it is because you do not have enough stomach juices to break down your nutrients. Betaine HCl and glutamic acid will eliminate upset tummy.

5. Ensure your supplement program is complete. Women need a full complement of vitamins, minerals, cofactors, herbs and essential fats every day. If you are only taking a couple of vitamins, you will not gain all the benefits.

6. Look out for "magic" pills. If your multivitamin with minerals only fits into one tablet you won't be taking the types, amounts or quality of nutrients sufficient to make a difference in your health. The best quality nutrients are sometimes bulky, making the one-a-day impossible to deliver an effective dose.

7. Make taking your essential nutrients a healthy habit. If you are like many women, you buy nutrients but forget to take them. Either put all your supplements for the day in a zip lock bag or look for a formula that comes in a handy packet that can be popped into your handbag to be taken at work during lunch.

Your multi-nutrient formula should *never*:

■ contain iron, as too much iron can increase your risk of heart disease and cancer. Only those with true iron deficiency confirmed by a serum ferritin, should take iron supplements if your physician recommends it. *See* Anemia for more information.

■ have the wrong ratio of calcium to magnesium. Clinical research on humans has proven that approximately twice the calcium as magnesium is required. Research shows that taking more magnesium than calcium can actually suppress calcium levels and increase bone loss by decreasing the production of the hormone calcitonin. Femmessentials and Multi-Essentials contain a 2:1 ratio of calcium to magnesium to ensure that your calcitonin, important for absorption and retention of calcium, functions optimally. 1000 mg of calcium citrate/chelate and 500 mg of magnesium citrate/chelate are necessary for female bone health—from teenagers to seniors. Make sure your multinutrient formula also contains vitamin D.

■ lack alkalinizing minerals because they are essential for proper pH balance in the body.

If your multi-nutrients are not of the highest quality, you won't see the results. Please make sure whichever multi-nutrient combination you take meets the following high standards:

NUTRITION CHART

RECOMMENDED NUTRIENTS (form)	NUTRIENT ACTION	FOOD SOURCES	DAILY AMOUNT
VITAMIN A (Palmitate)	Supports immune function, eye health, improves wound healing, anti-cancer, beautiful skin, fertility, bone support and cell function.	egg yolks, liver, kidney, full fat milk and cheese, butter, cod liver oil and halibut oil	5000 IU
BETA CAROTENE (Provitamin A)	Improves infection fighting, night vision, skin, immune function, thyroid activity, respiratory health, normalizes blood glucose and insulin.	dark green, red and deep yellow-orange vegetables	15 000 IU
VITAMIN B1 (Thiamine hydrochloride)	Enhances energy and vitality, reduces the effects of aging, improves cardiovascular and mental function.	brewer's yeast, organ meats, brown rice, soybeans and peanuts	60 mg
VITAMIN B2 (Riboflavin)	Enhances metabolism, improves vision.	green leafy vegetables, soybeans, whole grains, almonds, organ meats, poultry and eggs	60 mg
NIACIN	Improves cardiovascular health, lowers cholesterol, aids adrenal and hormone production, calms nervous system, boosts energy.	avocados, whole grains, legumes, eggs, milk, fish, organ meats, peanuts and poultry	30 mg
NIACINAMIDE	Improves cardiovascular health, aids adrenal and hormone production, calms nervous system, boosts energy.	avocados, whole grains, legumes, eggs, milk, fish, organ meats, peanuts and poultry	30 mg
VITAMIN B6 (Pyridoxal –5– phosphate)	Supports immune function, reduces homocysteine, improves cardiovascular function, mental clarity, reduces symptoms of menopause and PMS.	cantaloupe, bananas, cruciferous vegetables, eggs, organ meats, whole grains and saltwater fish	60 mg
VITAMIN B12 (Methylcobalamin)	Supports nerves, needed to prevent anemia.	meats, fish, eggs and cheese (vegans and vegetarians need supplementation)	1000 mcg
D-PANTOTHENIC ACID (Calcium pantothenate)	Supports the adrenal glands, increases energy, helps you better handle stressful situations, reduces cellulite.	organ meats, fish, poultry, legumes, mushrooms, nuts, eggs, strawberries, oranges and cruciferous vegetables	250 mg
FOLIC ACID	Reduces birth defects, enhances digestion, helps prevent anemia, elevates serotonin in the brain, needed for cellular repair.	asparagus, citrus fruit, lentils, legumes, whole grains, salmon, organ meats, beets and green leafy vegetables	1 mg

RECOMMENDED NUTRIENTS (form)	NUTRIENT ACTION	FOOD SOURCES	DAILY AMOUNT
BIOTIN	Improves energy production and healthy hair and skin; reduces muscle pain and depression; stops inflamed, sore tongue; reduces nausea and vomiting.	kidney, liver and organ meats, mushrooms, wheat bran and whole grains, eggs, nuts, legumes, cauliflower, sardines and salmon	500 mcg
VITAMIN C (Calcium ascorbate)	Improves cardiovascular and immune function, important for diabetes, anti aging, antiviral, antibacterial, enhances glutathione for detoxification.	vine-ripened fruits and vegetables, cruciferous vegetables, black currants, citrus fruits, sweet red and green peppers	600 mg
VITAMIN E (100% natural) (d-alpha tocopheryl succinate)	Improves cardiovascular function, reduces the effects of stress, improves skin and hair, reduces cramps and PMS symptoms, protects against arthritis, macular degeneration and diabetes and is an anti-aging nutrient and antioxidant.	dark green leafy vegetables, and cold pressed organic nut seed oils, butter, wheat germ, egg yolks, avocado, salmon, tuna, shrimp, lobster and soy	200 IU

LIPOTROPIC FACTORS

CHOLINE BITARTRATE	Supports brain function, nervous system and improves liver activity.	egg yolks, legumes and whole grains	100 mg
INOSITOL	Supports nervous system and cell function.	egg yolk, legumes and whole grains	100 mg

MINERALS

MAGNESIUM (Citrate/Chelate)	Promotes healthy nervous system, prevents bone loss and diabetes, supports muscle function.	tofu, whole grains, green leafy vegetables, nuts and seeds and legumes	250 mg
POTASSIUM (Citrate)	Protects against hypertension and stroke, promotes clear thinking.	kiwi, bananas, potatoes, lean poultry, fish, legumes, seeds and whole grains	100 mg
MANGANESE (Citrate)	Supports blood sugar control, thyroid activity, and energy metabolism, important for skin, hair and nails.	whole grains, nuts and green leafy vegetables	15 mg
ZINC (Citrate)	Protects against hair loss, improves skin and nails, supports joint and tissues and is essential for thymus function.	red meat, oysters, nuts and peanut butter, wheat bran and germ	15 mg
IODINE (Kelp)	Regulates estrogen in breast tissue, protects against fibrocystic breasts, important for reproductive function and is critical for thyroid hormone.	seafood, kelp and dulse	0.3 mg

RECOMMENDED NUTRIENTS (form)	NUTRIENT ACTION	FOOD SOURCES	DAILY AMOUNT
CHROMIUM (Chelate)	Stabilizes glucose levels, enhances energy and metabolism, important for weight loss, lowers cholesterol and triglycerides.	whole grains, liver, cheese, nuts and peanuts	200 mcg
SELENIUM (Chelate)	Improves immune function, important for cellular repair and has anti-cancer properties.	Brazil nuts	100 mcg
VANADIUM (Citrate)	Improves blood sugar control and metabolism.	pepper, dill, radishes, eggs, organic nut and seed oils, buckwheat and oats	75 mcg
MOLYBDENUM (Citrate)	Supports detoxification, anti-cancer, important for iron metabolism.	whole grains, dark green leafy vegetables and legumes	25 mcg

OTHER NUTRIENTS	ACTIONS	D/AMOUNT
CITRUS BIOFLAVONOIDS extract 4:1	Protects against carcinogenic estrogens, stimulates weight loss, protects against allergies, promotes circulation, reduces the risk of osteoporosis, antibacterial and anti-cancer.	100 mg
BETAINE HCl	Aids digestion of fats, proteins and minerals.	50 mg
FENNEL EXTRACT 4:1 (Foeniculium vulgare)	Soothes the digestive tract, aids digestion and eases PMS symptoms.	50 mg
GLUTAMIC ACID HCl	Improves digestion, reduces the risk of kidney stones and is for gut health.	50 mg
GRAPESEED PHYTOSOME™	Protects blood vessels and prevents arteriosclerosis, anti-allergy, anti-aging and stops varicose veins.	10 mg
GREEN TEA PHYTOSOME™	Burns fat and increases metabolism, anti-cancer and detoxifies carcinogenic estrogens.	10 mg
INDOLE-3-CARBINOL	Detoxifies carcinogenic estrogens, anti-cancer, reduces the risk of breast, ovarian and HPV-induced cervical cancer.	5 mg
LUTEIN (Tagetes erecta)	Improves vision and is important for those with macular degeneration.	1 mg

Balanced Essential Fatty Acid Complex

NUTRIENTS	ACTIONS	D/AMOUNT
EVENING PRIMROSE OIL (non-GMO)	Supports normal cardiovascular health. Promotes glowing skin, hair and nails.	1000 mg
ORGANIC FLAX OIL (non-GMO)	Balances hormones, aids optimal digestion, important for cellular and membrane repair, reduces menstrual and menopausal symptoms, reduces inflammation, improves mood.	1600 mg

Bone Support Nutrients

NUTRIENTS	ACTIONS	FOOD SOURCES	D/AMOUNT
CALCIUM (Citrate/Chelate)	Prevents bone loss, improves nerve function, enhances energy production, supports healthy cardiovascular function.	sea vegetables, kale, green leafy vegetables, cruciferous vegetables, sesame and sunflower seeds, brazil nuts, almonds, tofu	1000 mg
VITAMIN D3	Improves calcium absorption, prevents osteoporosis, reduces muscle cramps and twitching, essential for proper thyroid function, improves skin condition.	egg yolks, cod liver oil, fatty fish, fortified milk products	400 IU
SILICON (Horsetail)	Strengthens bone structure, connective tissues, prevents arteriosclerosis.	whole grains, well water, bottled mineral water, fresh vegetables	4 mg
MAGNESIUM (Citrate)	Prevents bone loss and diabetes, supports muscle function.	tofu, whole grains, green leafy vegetables, nuts, seeds and legumes	250 mg

Make a commitment to do one important thing for yourself–take your essential nutrients every day. You can either buy the supplements mentioned above separately or in packets. FemmEssentials by Preferred Nutrition in Canada or MultiEssentials from Natural Factors in the U.S. are the two brands that I developed for myself and my daughters.

APPENDIX B:

WOMEN'S HEALTH SELF-ASSESSMENT QUESTIONNAIRES

■ Stress Test to Determine Adrenal Health

Lifestyle

Give yourself 4 points for each situation that applies to you; 3 if it only applies occasionally.

___ I am a single mother.

___ I am a university student.

___ I am in an unhappy marriage.

___ I live with an alcoholic or drug abuser.

___ I work shift work.

___ I like my job, but have too much work to do.

___ I like my job, but my boss is too demanding.

___ I shop to make myself feel better.

___ I work too much and don't have enough play time.

___ I don't eat regularly (more than 4-5 hours between meals).

___ I smoke, drink alcohol or consume more than 2 cups of caffeinated beverages (coffee, tea, colas, sodas) daily.

___ My family and friends are not supportive of the things I do.

___ I have friends who take but never give.

Emotions

Rate your negative emotions on a scale of 1 to 4; 1 is for feelings you have on occasion, 4 is for emotions you experience frequently.

___ I am worried about paying my bills this month.

___ I look at myself in the mirror and think negative thoughts.

___ I am lonely.

___ I dislike my job.

___ I am always trying to please everyone.
___ I have feelings of guilt or anger.
___ I am afraid of failure.
___ I have feelings of anxiety or low moods.
___ I feel trapped or that I can't cope sometimes.
___ I get angry with myself.

Physical Symptoms

Give yourself 4 points for symptoms you have frequently; 3 for those that occur often, 2 for occasional symptoms, and 1 for symptoms you have had in the past.

___ I am exhausted, but keep going.
___ My stomach feels like it has butterflies.
___ I crave sugar.
___ I am sick more than three times a year.
___ I lack sexual desire.
___ I am tired all the time.

Total Score: _____

How did you score?

If you scored from 1 to 15, you need to find more balance in your life.

If you scored from 16 to 30, you know you have to make some changes. You are still coping, but you are at risk of adrenal exhaustion.

If you scored over 30, you know you are over the top and need to adopt strategies to reduce your risk of stress-related disease.

While many of the stressors mentioned above may not seem to be stress promoters, these kinds of issues provide constant, low-grade stress that keeps you in that state of unease that leads to adrenal exhaustion. *See* Adrenal Exhaustion for more information.

■ Breast Health Self-Assessment

For every situation that applies to you, give yourself the numbers of points indicated on the right.

___ I have not had children and am under 25.	1
___ I have not had children and am 25 to 35.	2
___ I have no children, and don't intend to have any.	3
___ I did not breastfeed.	2
___ I took birth control pills during teens or early 20s. (A few months use may increase risk of breast cancer by 30 percent. Ten years use may double it.)	3
___ I have taken or am taking HRT (Premarin, Provera, Prempro).	3
___ I had regular mammograms before menopause.	2
___ I don't exercise three times per week.	2
___ I have had depression where tricyclic anti-depressants were prescribed. (studies showed increase in mammary tumors in rats)	2
___ I have breast implants. (causes breast trauma)	1
___ I had chest X-rays as a teenager or during my 20s.	2
___ I am exposed to Electric and Magnetic Fields (EMFs) due to excessive computer use, hair dryer use, or I live close to power lines.	1
___ I dye my hair with dark-coloured dyes. (a source of xenoestrogens)	2
___ I wear dry-cleaned clothing. (a source of xenoestrogens)	1
___ I use bleached sanitary products, e.g., tampons, pads. (a source of xenoestrogens)	2
___ I eat pesticide- and herbicide-laden foods.	3
___ I use nail polish that is not toluene or phthalate-free.	1
___ My periods started before age 12.	2
___ I had late onset menopause, starting after age 50.	2
___ I eat a diet high in animal fat, dairy and meat. (a source of xenoestrogens)	3
___ I smoke, with early or excessive use.	3
___ I drink alcohol, with early or excessive use.	3
___ I don't eat cruciferous vegetables. (These vegetables detoxify carcinogenic estrogens.)	3
___ I take cholesterol-lowering drugs, which deplete the body of Coexzyme Q10. (Co-Q10 protects against breast cancer.)	3

___ I am using anti-hypertensives for lowering high blood pressure. (Depletes Co-Q10)   **3**

___ I am using tranquilizers. (Studies show an increase in breast tumors if tranquilizers are used regularly.)   **2**

___ I am using ulcer medications. (Disrupts estrogen metabolism, which decreases good estrogen.)   **2**

___ I am overweight or obese. (fat stores estrogens)   **3**

___ I use or have used Flagyl for yeast infections. (Studies show an increase in mammary tumors in rats.)   **2**

___ A first degree relative (mother, sister or daughter) has had breast cancer.)   **1**

Total Score: _____

0-18	lower risk
19-35	moderate to high risk
35-65	high risk

See Breast Cancer for more information.

■ Osteoporosis Questionnaire

Choose the descriptor in each category that best describes you, and fill in the point value for that descriptor in the space to the right. You may choose more than one descriptor in categories marked with an asterisk.

If your total score is greater than 50, you are at significant risk for osteoporosis.

	Points	Score
• Frame Size		
___ Small-boned or petite	10	_____
___ Medium frame, very lean	5	_____
___ Medium frame, average or heavy build	0	_____
___ Large frame, very lean	5	_____
• Ethnic Background		
___ Caucasian	10	_____
___ Asian	10	_____
___ Other	0	_____

- Activity Level

How often do you walk briskly, jog, do aerobics or weight lifting, or perform hard physical labour for at least 30 minutes?

___ Seldom	30	_____
___ 1 to 2 times per week	20	_____
___ 3 to 4 times per week	5	_____
___ 5 or more times per week	0	_____

- Smoking

___ Smoke 10 or more cigarettes a day	20	_____
___ Smoke fewer than 10 cigarettes a day	10	_____
___ Quit smoking	5	_____
___ Never smoked	0	_____

- Personal Health Factors*

___ Family history of osteoporosis	20	_____
___ Long-term corticosteroid use	20	_____
___ Long-term anticonvulsant use	20	_____
___ Drink more than 3 glasses of alcohol per week	20	_____
___ Drink more than 1 cup of coffee per day	10	_____
___ Seldom get outside in the sun	10	_____
___ Have had ovaries removed	10	_____
___ Premature menopause	10	_____
___ Have had no children	10	_____

- Dietary Factors*

___ Consume more than 120 g meat per day	20	_____
___ Drink soft drinks regularly	20	_____
___ Consume 3 to 5 servings of vegetables per day	-10	_____
___ Take a calcium supplement	-10	_____
___ Consume a vegetarian diet	-10	_____

Total Score:_____

Adapted from *The Encyclopedia of Natural Medicine* by Michael T. Murray, N.D., and Joseph Pizzomo, N.D. (Prima Health)

See Osteoporosis for more information

■ Blood Sugar Problem Symptom List

To arrive at your final score, write:

0 beside symptoms you never or almost never experience

1 beside symptoms you occasionally have, but do not affect you severely

2 beside symptoms you occasionally have and that affect you severely

3 beside symptoms you experience frequently, but which do not affect you severely

4 beside symptoms you experience frequently and that affect you severely

___ Afternoon exhaustion

___ Allergies

___ Anxiety

___ Awaken after a few hours sleep hard to get back to sleep (insomnia)

___ Aware of breathing heavily

___ Blurred vision

___ "Butterfly stomach," cramps

___ Can't concentrate

___ Can't decide easily

___ Can't start in the morning without coffee

___ Can't work under pressure

___ Chronic indigestion

___ Cold hands or feet

___ Constantly hungry

___ Crave alcohol

___ Crave bread

___ Crave candy or coffee in the afternoons

___ Crave chocolate

___ Craving for sweets

___ Cry easily for no apparent reason

___ Depression

___ Dizziness

___ Eat when nervous

___ Fatigue, relieved by eating

___ Forgetfulness

___ Frequent urination

___ Get "shaky" if hungry

___ Headaches

___ Heart palpitations

___ Indecisiveness

___ Irritable before meals

___ Irritability (general)

___ Joint pain

___ Lack energy

___ Moodiness

___ Muscle pain and backache

___ Muscular twitching or cramps

___ Nervousness

___ Night urination

___ Noise or light sensitivity

___ Obesity

___ Peculiar breath or perspiration odor

___ Poor exercise tolerance

___ Premenstrual symptoms (PMS)

___ Reduced initiative

___ Restlessness

___ Sighing and yawning

___ Sleepy after meals

___ Sleepy during day

___ Sweating

___ Weakness

Total Score:_____

See Diabetes for more information

■ *Candida* Questionnaire

General History

Enter (3) if you answer "yes" to any of the following:

___ Have you taken tetracyclines (e.g., Minocin) for acne for one month or longer?

___ Have you taken, or do you take, antibiotics for infections more than four times per year?

___ Have you taken birth control pills for more than two years?

___ Have you taken birth control pills for six months to two years?

___ Have you taken prednisone or other cortisone-like drugs (e.g., asthma medication)?

___ Does the smell of perfume, tobacco or other odors or chemicals make you sick?

___ Do you crave sugars and breads?

Symptoms

Enter (1) if symptom is mild; (2) if moderate or frequent; (3) if severe or constant.

___ Experience vaginal discharge or irritation

___ Experience frequent bladder infections or incontinence

___ Experience premenstrual syndrome or fluid retention

___ Have difficulty getting pregnant

___ Have frequent infections (sinus, lung, colds, etc.)

___ Have allergies to foods or environmental substances

___ Feel worse on rainy and snowy days, around molds or musty basements

___ Experience feelings of anxiety and/or irritability

___ Have insomnia

___ Experience gas and bloating

___ Experience constipation or diarrhea

___ Have bad breath

___ Have a difficult time concentrating; feel "spacey"

___ Experience muscle weakness or painful joints

___ Have nasal congestion

___ Feel pressure behind or irritation in my eyes

___ Have frequent headaches

___ Generally "not feeling well" without an explanation or diagnosis

___ Have thyroid problems

___ Have muscle aches or weakness

___ Total Score from both sections

Scoring:

50 or less indicates mild *Candida*

50 to 90 indicates moderate *Candida*

90 to 120 indicates severe *Candida*

See Vaginal Yeast Infections for prevention and treatment of
***Candida albicans* overgrowth.**

■ Symptoms and their associated organ system

Many of the following symptoms, while commonly attributed to perimenopause or menopause, are actually associated with adrenal dysfunction (A), thyroid dysfunction (T), liver congestion (L) and *Candida*/intestinal problems (C).

- Acceleration of the aging process – overnight wrinkles appear (T, A)
- Anxiety or panic attacks (A, C)
- Bloating and indigestion, gas (T, C)
- Increase in blood pressure or cholesterol (A, T, L)
- Bone pain (often associated with osteoporosis/osteopenia) (A)
- Inability to breathe deeply (air hunger) (A)
- "Crawly" skin sensations, especially of the lower limbs (restless leg syndrome) (A, L)
- Low energy (A, T, L, C)
- Increased facial hair, particularly around the chin and upper lip (A, T, L)
- Heart palpitations (T, A)
- Hot feet, worse in bed (L)
- Hot flushes and/or night sweats (L, C)
- Insomnia or interrupted sleep (A, T, C, L)
- Itching around the vaginal area, with or without discharge (C)
- Joint and muscle aches and pains (L, T)
- Diminished libido, painful intercourse (A, T)
- Lightheadedness, dizzy spells, vertigo (A)
- Memory problems, brain fog (A, C)
- Mood changes, depression, irritability or anger (L, A)
- Migraine headaches (L, C)
- New food or environmental sensitivities or allergies (C, L, A)
- Urinary incontinence (worse with coughing or laughing) (C)
- Vaginal or urinary tract infections (C)
- Weight gain, usually around or on the abdomen, hips, and breasts (T)

APPENDIX C:

Diagnostic Tests and Types of Treatments

BREAST HEALTH

Breast Self-examinations

Breast Self-Examination (BSE) does not prevent cancer, but many women discover abnormalities in their breasts during regular home testing. Perform the exam the day after your period ends each month. Or, for non-menstruating women, pick the same day each month. Follow these directions to perform your self-examination:

- Lie down and put a pillow under your right shoulder. Place your right arm behind your head.
- Use the finger pads of your three middle fingers on your left hand to feel for lumps or thickening in your right breast. Your finger pads are the top third of each finger. Press firmly enough to know how your breast feels. Learn what your breast feels like most of the time. A firm ridge in the lower curve of each breast is normal. You can either make a circle or move your fingers up and down.
- Move around the breast the same way each time you do the examination so you are aware of any changes.
- Switch the pillow to your other shoulder, and repeat with your left breast, using the right-hand finger pads.
- Repeat the examination of both breasts while standing, with one arm behind your head. The upright position makes it easier to check the upper and outer parts of the breasts (toward your armpit). (You may want to do the standing part of the BSE while you are in the shower. Some breast changes can be felt more easily when your skin is wet and soapy.)
- Check your breasts for any dimpling of the skin, changes in the nipples, redness, or swelling while standing in front of a mirror right after your BSE each month.

Remember that most women have lumps or lumpy areas in their breasts, so don't panic if you find a lump. Report any changes to your doctor. A clinical examination is very much the same as BSE, except that a trained professional may discover abnormalities that you may find insignificant. Both examinations are considered important in detecting cancers early.

Mammogram

Every October, during Breast Cancer Month, national campaigns encourage you to "prevent" breast cancer by having your annual mammogram. A mammogram does not prevent breast cancer. It is a diagnostic tool, albeit, as we are discovering, not the most effective one.

Danish researchers reviewed seven randomized, controlled mammogram trials that supported the benefits of mammography in reducing the rate of death from breast cancer. They found that, out of the seven trials, five were so flawed they could not be considered useful; the two remaining trials also had problems. Researchers determined that mammograms had no effect on reducing deaths due to breast cancer. Published in the *Journal of the National Cancer Institute (JNCI)*, a more recent study that followed over 40,000 women between the ages of 50 and 59 found mammograms do not reduce death rates from breast cancer any better than a simple breast exam.

Mammogram Concerns

The chance of receiving a false positive from mammography is substantial (meaning you have been diagnosed with a cancer when there is none), according to the *JNCI*. Women in their 40s are at higher risk of false positives due to dense breast tissue. Women who have been taking hormone replacement therapy (estrogen and progestins) have much denser breast tissue, making it difficult to detect abnormal tissue.

A study published in the *Journal of the American Medical Association* found that women age 70 and older had little to no benefit from regular mammograms. *The Lancet* reported that breast compression, which occurs during mammography, may cause tumors to rupture, spreading cancer cells.

The safety of repeated ionizing radiation from mammograms has been questioned amid concerns that it may increase the risk of breast cancer.

What's a woman to do? Researchers reported to the 39th Annual Meeting of the American Society of Oncology that Magnetic Resonance Imaging (MRI) offered, by far, the highest sensitivity for diagnosing breast cancer—with the lowest rate of unnecessary biopsies. An MRI uses magnetic energy, not X-rays, to view the breast tissue. They found that MRIs provided 96.1 percent accuracy in reporting positive results, compared to mammography (42.8 percent accurate) and ultrasound

(41 percent accurate). We need to insist on better detection methods. Ask your doctor about MRI as an alternative to mammogram. Women should have a baseline breast MRI performed at 40 and then start annual MRIs at age 50.

Thermography

Another promising screening tool is thermography, which is less expensive and sometimes easier to obtain than an MRI.

In order to survive, a cancer tumor has to develop a supply of nutrients. In the early stages, it does this by stealing blood supply and nutrients from nearby cells. This process of angiogenesis continues until the blood cells form tiny capillaries that reach the tumor and start the supply of oxygen and nutrients that fuels rapid growth of the cancer. As the cancer grows, it forms a lump that can be felt during a clinical exam or seen on mammogram, but, long before a lump is felt, heat is produced that can be detected via thermography.

All of this activity within the breast causes changes in the surface temperature of the skin. Thermography, or infrared imaging, is a non-invasive, painless technique that can indicate breast abnormalities, including benign tumors, cancer, fibrocystic breast disease, mastitis or other health issues, at very early stages. In fact, sensitive thermographic equipment is able to detect potential cancers at the stage where blood is pooling near the tumor site. Although thermography is not able to pinpoint the exact location of a tumor, it is extremely useful as a predictor of future cancer risks and, combined with other tests, could help to prevent invasive tumor growth.

During the procedure, a woman sits in a cool room, and removes her clothing from the waist up. Although her skin temperature will drop and blood activity will slow, cancerous and pre-cancerous cells are highly active and operate independent of the nervous system. As a result, these areas will continue to produce heat that will be captured by the sensitive infrared camera. Thermography is effective for detecting angiogenesis in dense breast tissue, so it is suitable for young women as well. Annual thermograms should become part of every woman's breast-health protection strategy especially if you have decided not to have a mammogram or MRI.

REPRODUCTIVE HEALTH

PAP test

A Papanicolaou Test (PAP) should be performed annually after age 18 or before, if the woman is sexually active, and/or taking the birth control pill. The PAP test, also called the PAP smear, is a diagnostic test used to detect abnormal cell growth on the cervix. During this test a speculum is inserted into the vagina and the cells of the cervix are gently scraped off to be examined. This test does not hurt.

Cancer of the cervix develops when the cells on the surface of the cervix divide and grow uncontrollably. It takes years for this cancer to develop and during this time, normal cells change. This change can be detected by a PAP test. We call these abnormal cells which have not become cancerous *dysplasia*. Mild dysplasia can develop into severe dysplasia, and then cancer, if left untreated.

HPV and abnormal PAP tests: Human papilloma virus, a virus that causes the growth of warts, is often associated with cancer of the cervix and/or dysplasia, chronic urinary tract infections, vaginosis and vaginitis. HPV is considered the most common sexually transmitted disease. It should not be confused with sexual promiscuity; women who have had the same partner for 20 years can contract HPV. Women who have abnormal PAP tests should also be tested for HPV. Of the more than 70 HPV types that have been identified, about 30 infect the cervix.

More often an abnormal PAP test is a result of hormonal changes (women on the Pill have a higher rate of abnormal PAP tests), menopause, douching, infection, *Candida* overgrowth and irritation or inflammation.

Classification of PAP test results

There are two classification methods commonly in use today: the Bethesda System and the CIN Grading System.

Bethesda System:
- ASCUS (atypical squamous cells of undetermined significance) – Borderline, some abnormal cells
- LGSIL (low-grade squamous intraepithelial lesions) – Mild dysplasia and cellular changes associated with HPV

- HGSIL (high-grade squamous intraepithelial lesions) – Moderate to severe dysplasia, precancerous lesions and carcinoma in-situ (preinvasive cancer that involves only the surface cells)

CIN Grading System: CIN stands for Cervical Intraepithelial Neoplasia. This system grades the degree of cell abnormality numerically.

Atypia – correlates with ASCUS
CIN I – mild dysplasia and correlates with LGSIL
CIN II – moderate dysplasia and correlates with HGSIL
CIN III – severe dysplasia and correlates with HGSIL
Carcinoma in-situ
Cervical cancer

To find out how to normalize PAP smears, *see* Cervical Dysplasia.

Ultrasound

Any type of abnormal bleeding or pelvic pain should be evaluated with a pelvic ultrasound (sonography). An ultrasound scan uses high-frequency sound waves that are sent to the body part being examined; these waves are reflected back and displayed on a monitor screen. Pelvic sonography is used to examine the pelvic cavity, ovaries, uterus, endometrium, fallopian tubes, bladder, kidneys and ureters. It is also used to evaluate infertility and to monitor fetal health during pregnancy. Pelvic ultrasounds can be performed vaginally (vaginal ultrasound) or externally, on the belly. Women are asked to consume plenty of water before the procedure so the sound waves can bounce off the bladder for the best possible image.

TREATMENT

Hysterectomy

A hysterectomy is the surgical removal of the uterus, the organ that holds a baby during pregnancy. With over 772,000 operations annually in the U.S. and 60,000 in Canada, hysterectomy is the second most common surgery performed on women, after cesarean section. Before the age of 60, one in three American women will have had a hysterectomy. In Canada, the number is closer to 37 percent. The main reason for hysterectomy is uterine fibroids, which result in heavy periods and anemia, while endometriosis is the second leading cause. Be sure to read the appropriate sections of this book for alternative treatments for these conditions. (See Myomectomy and Uterine Artery Embolization in this section; see also Uterine Fibroids and Endometriosis.)

About 16 percent of hysterectomies are due to uterine prolapse. This occurs when the uterus relocates from its normal position and falls further into the vagina. Prolapse occurs due to weakened ligaments and supportive tissues that frequently result from childbirth, lack of exercise, hormone imbalance at menopause (particularly testosterone deficiency) or obesity. Before considering removal of the uterus, women should try other options including exercise, Kegal exercises or the use of a pessary. Kegel exercises involve squeezing the muscles of the pelvic floor, vagina and buttock muscles. Squeeze, hold and release several times per day. Practice Kegal exercises while urinating. Start and stop the urine stream to improve bladder control while improving internal pelvic muscles.

A pessary is a plastic ring that is inserted into the vagina to support the uterus. Alternatively, less traumatic surgery can tighten the muscles and ligaments around the uterus to help hold it in place. In about ten percent of cases, hysterectomies are performed due to cancers of the reproductive tract.

Many believe that the uterus is a useless organ after a woman has finished having babies. Evidence shows that the uterus plays a role in immune function—it produces the prostaglandins responsible for a variety of physiological functions. The uterus helps in prevention of cardiovascular disease through the production of prostacyclin, which prevents blood clots. The uterus also secretes a small amount of estrogen. Women who have had hysterectomies also appear to be at increased risk of osteoporosis and osteoarthritis. Hysterectomy also impacts libido: in some women the removal of the uterus causes an abrupt end to her sex drive. In fact, particularly in the case of hysterectomy due to prolapsed uterus, research shows that 50 percent of hysterectomies end sexual intercourse permanently. The reason for this can be due to the surgeon damaging nerves or inhibiting blood flow to the clitoris or pelvic region.

Surgical Risks: Any surgery has risks, but women who are obese, or who have high blood pressure, diabetes or other chronic conditions are at increased risk. Complications of surgery include damage and scarring of surrounding internal organs such as the ureters (tubes which carry urine from the bladder to the kidneys), the rectum and the bladder. Deep vein thrombosis involves blood clots that form in the legs but break free and move to the lungs where they can get trapped, causing a potentially fatal embolism. Women who have hysterectomies before menopause may suddenly experience severe menopause symptoms. (*See* Menopause)

Types of Hysterectomy: With the exception of cancer treatment, hysterectomy should only be performed after you have exhausted all of the options discussed in this book. If you must have a hysterectomy, discuss all of your concerns and evaluate all your choices before proceeding. Also, find an skilled surgeon.

■ **Complete or Total Hysterectomy:** Also known as a pan-hysterectomy, this is the most commonly performed operation. It involves the removal of the entire uterus, with or without the ovaries. Most women think a total hysterectomy means the removal of the ovaries, but that is false.

■ **Partial Hysterectomy:** Also known as a supracervical hysterectomy, this surgery leaves leaves the cervix and the ovaries in place; only the uterus is removed.

■ **Bilateral Salpingo-oophorectomy:** This procedure removes the ovaries and fallopian tubes on both sides of the uterus. This can be done with or without the removal of the uterus.

■ **Radical Hysterectomy:** As its name implies, this procedure removes the uterus, the cervix, the ovaries, the upper part of the vagina and other supporting tissues.

Procedure: A hysterectomy can be performed either with an abdominal incision or through the vagina. During an abdominal hysterectomy, the surgery is performed through an incision in the abdomen. Surgeons may be able to use a bikini-line incision just above the pubic bone, but often the incision is made vertically.

Vaginal hysterectomies are performed through the vagina. In this form of surgery the cervix is removed as well. Vaginal hysterectomy patients have shorter recovery times because there is no abdominal incision.

LAPAROSCOPY
Laparoscopically assisted vaginal hysterectomies involve the use of a small viewing tube (a laparoscope) through an incision in the abdominal wall. Laparoscopy,

where an incision is made in the bellybutton, is done for many types of female conditions, including the diagnosis or removal of endometriosis, ovarian cysts or to evaluate unexplained pelvic pain. During a laparoscopy, usually a very tiny incision is made in the bellybutton and another at the side of the abdomen and one just above the pubic bone. One is for the laparoscope and the others for the surgical instruments. The abdomen is filled with air for ease of viewing.

MICROWAVE ENDOMETRIAL ABLATION (MEA)

Microwave ablation is currently being studied by the medical community as an alternative to surgery for a variety of conditions including heart surgeries as well as a method of treating liver tumors, prostate cancer and breast cancer. In fact, a study published in 2003 showed that microwave ablation was able to halt the growth of early-stage breast tumors in 68 percent of women tested. While still in its infancy as a treatment for breast cancer, microwave endometrial ablation has gained wide acceptance as an alternative to hysterectomy for women with fibroids and menorrhagia (heavy menstrual bleeding).

MEA uses high-frequency microwave energy to heat and destroy the lining of the uterus, or the endometrium. Before microwave endometrial ablation is performed, women are given hormones to further thicken the uterine lining. Then, to prevent perforating the uterus, a woman typically undergoes an ultrasound to determine the minimal thickness of the uterine wall. During the procedure, the cervix is dilated and the doctor inserts a wand-like device into the uterine cavity. The surgeon then moves the applicator around the uterus to destroy the lining. The temperature of the device is strictly monitored, and has an automatic shut-off valve if temperature rises too high. The procedure is carried out under local or general anesthetic and typically takes less than ten minutes to complete. The uterus no longer functions as it used to and pregnancy cannot occur once this treatment has been completed.

MEA has a shorter recovery time than hysterectomy, and the uterus is not removed from the body. Similar to hysterectomy, MEA is not an option for women who are considering pregnancy.

Myomectomy

Uterine fibroids affect a vast number of women. Many exhibit no symptoms, while others have pain or abnormal bleeding. (*See* Uterine Fibroids) Although hysterectomy is often the first choice to deal with the problem, a less invasive procedure called myomectomy surgically removes the fibroids but leaves the uterus intact. A method called hysteroscopic resection can remove fibroids located inside the uterus through the cervix without the need for an incision. Some fibroids lodged partially in the wall of the uterus and partially in the uterine cavity can also be removed using this procedure. Laparoscopy can often treat fibroids on the outside of the uterus. Larger fibroids can be removed through abdominal surgery, which has a healing time similar to a hysterectomy, but again, leaves the uterus in place. Myomectomy is the recommended treatment for infertility caused by the uterine fibroids in women still wishing to conceive.

Uterine Artery Embolization

A relatively new procedure, uterine artery embolization (UAE) is used to cut off the blood supply to the arteries that feed the fibroid. Small particles of polyvinyl alcohol about the size of a grain of sand are injected into the arteries, and the blockage causes the uterine fibroid to shrink in size or die and symptoms improve. The particles are locked into the vessels so they do not travel through the body. This procedure is not readily available in all communities and there have been reports of emergency hysterectomies having to be performed as a side effect of UAE. Because the long-term effects are not yet known, women considering pregnancy are not suitable candidates for UAE.

THYROID HEALTH

Thyroid Stimulating Hormone (TSH) thyroid test
Laboratory Tests: TSH, T3 and T4. The normal levels for the TSH test are so broadly defined that most patients with functional problems are not clinically diagnosable. Yet it takes very little change in the pituitary stimulating hormone TSH to cause dramatic changes in thyroid function. It is a mystery why the allopathic definition of the normal range for TSH is so wide, given the extreme sensitivity of the thyroid to even minute variations in TSH levels.

Many people suffer with mild or sub-clinical low thyroid function. Their thyroid stimulating hormone (the hormone that stimulates the thyroid to make thyroid hormones) is greater than 2.0 IU/ml but less than the 5.5 IU/ml level indicative of hypothyroidism. As such, these people contend with the many symptoms of low thyroid function, but are not being treated with medication. For more information on Thyroid function, see Thyroid. For additional information on T3, please refer to the work of Dr. E. D. Wilson, *Wilson's Syndrome: The Miracle of Feeling Well.*

Thyroid Basal Temperature Home test

Monitoring your basal temperature is the most sensitive and accurate way to evaluate thyroid function; it is also the simplest and least expensive. The thyroid sets the thermostat for the body and regulates the rate of metabolism in nearly all of the cells. Therefore, the most reliable window on thyroid function is the basic body temperature, or basal temperature. Some health care practitioners call basal temperature the axillary temperature because it is measured in the armpit. It is measured at the same time every day—as soon as you wake up in the morning, before arising.

LOW THYROID HOME TEST

Your basal body temperature, meaning the temperature of your body at rest, is the most sensitive test of thyroid function. Note: Menstruating women must perform the test on the second, third and fourth days of menstruation. Men and postmenopausal women can perform the test any time.

- Take the test as soon as you wake up because it is important to take your temperature after you have had adequate rest.
- Before going to sleep, if you are not using a digital thermometer shake a regular thermometer to below the 95 degree mark and place it by your bed (ready to be used in the morning).
- Immediately upon waking, before you get out of bed, place the thermometer in your armpit (hold for a count of 10 if you are using a regular thermometer). Hold your elbow close to your side to keep the thermometer in place.
- Read and record the temperature and date.
- Repeat the test for three mornings (preferably at the same time every day).
- A reading between 97.6 and 98.2 degrees F is normal. Readings below 97.6 may indicate hypothyroidism.